Nurses, Gender and Sexuality

Nursing Today is a series that looks critically yet constructively at the work of nursing and the needs of nurses. Already published in this series is *The Politics of Nursing* and *Stress and Self-awareness: a Guide for Nurses*.

Nursing Today

Nurses, Gender and Sexuality

Jan Savage

Heinemann Nursing
London

Heinemann Medical Books
22 Bedford Square
London WC1B 3HH

ISBN 0–433–03491–2

© Jan Savage, 1987

First published 1987

British Library Cataloguing-in-Publication Data
Savage, Jan
    Nurses, gender and sexuality.—(Nursing
    today).
    1. Nurse and patient   2. Sick—Sexual
    behavior
    I. Title   II. Series
    610.73′06′99   RT86.3

    ISBN 0–433–03491–2

Typeset by Eta Services Ltd, Beccles
and printed in Great Britain by Biddles Ltd, Guildford

Contents

To Benjamin Feder and to the memory of Norah Prince.

Preface

The origins of this book date back to the time when I was a student on a gynaecological nursing course. A number of patients asked me how treatment might affect their sexuality—in particular their future sex lives—and I was unable to answer their questions. Turning to other nurses and nurse tutors for advice I was met by the kind of embarrassed silence which I was to find widespread within nursing. My first response was to collect together whatever material about gynaecology I could find and make it accessible to nurses working in this field (see Savage 1982). But it became clear that lack of information was only one part of the problem: the other was the uneasiness nurses experienced in coping with the entire issue of sexuality. This book examines the reasons for their disquiet. It questions what can reasonably be asked of nurses in terms of incorporating sexuality into nursing care, and hopes to offer reassurance to nurses who are struggling against the unrealistic expectations of their mentors. This book does not aim to provide all the answers, but instead to provoke discussion of the issues surrounding sexuality that have remained more or less taboo within nursing.

There are many people I should like to thank for their help in writing this book. First I would like to acknowledge the importance of the 'Gang of Three'—a study group which began several years ago. I should like to thank the other two members, Angie Cotter and Karen Greenwood, not only for the many discussions we have had on the issue of sexuality but also for their encouragement and support throughout all stages of this book. I hope they know how much I have valued this. They are, of course, deeply implicated in any mistakes I have made!

Secondly, I must state my appreciation to the staff of the Department of Anthropology at the London School of Economics, who were prepared to take me on as an undergraduate when no-one else would consider a nursing qualification equal to A levels. Through the study of the different meanings given to sexuality and gender, anthropology helped challenge some of my own culturally based notions about sexuality, especially its natural-ness, and has strongly influenced the stance I take in this book.

I must also thank all the nurses who spoke to me of their feelings and experiences. I am profoundly grateful for their help and openness. I was repeatedly struck by their integrity and goodwill despite the many difficulties they faced. As promised, they shall remain anonymous, although it is a sad reflection of the *modus operandi* within nursing that this should be felt necessary.

In addition I thank all those who have shown interest, offered support, listened, or taken time to make comments. In particular I thank Michelle Davies, Ted and Marika Feder, Julia James, Sarah Leyland, Greg Lucas, Frank Prince, Sally Redfern, Jane Salvage, the staff of the Thomas Guy and Lewisham School of Nursing, Jenny Thompson, Carrol Walsh, Richard Wells, Anne Woollett and Nancy Worcester.

Finally, a very special word of thanks to Gene Feder for his unfailing interest and encouragement.

Jan Savage
1987

Introduction: links between nursing, gender and sexuality

As nursing moves towards a recognition of the patient as a whole person rather than a diseased organ or a clutch of symptoms, an acknowledgement of the patient's sexuality becomes increasingly important. This is particularly the case if sexuality is understood to be concerned with all aspects of the individual, not just with their genitalia.

There are many signs that sexuality is receiving greater acknowledgement within nursing. Nurse education is attempting to incorporate issues of sexuality into the curriculum. The nursing press is less wary of publishing articles concerned with sexuality or sexual health, and books on these subjects are multiplying. At first glance it appears nursing has taken the patient's sexuality to its heart. But a second look shows that this has only really happened at a theoretical level; the intention to help the patient express his or her sexuality is rarely translated into action. In practice the issue is largely evaded.

One major reason for this is the way in which sexuality is defined by many nursing theorists. We are told that sexuality is a 'biopsychosocial phenomenon', a 'powerful and purposeful aspect of human nature'; in effect, we are told very little. Definitions of sexuality are vague almost to the point of meaninglessness and this vagueness camouflages considerable confusion. Sexuality is understood by some only to mean sexual intercourse. Alternatively, the term may be given a broader interpretation, emphasising the non-erotic aspects of sexuality at the expense of the erotic. Occasionally sexuality is used to refer to attitudes, characteristics and behaviour which are, within a particular culture, thought to accompany biological maleness or femaleness—in other words, gender. Gender, however, represents only one aspect of sexuality.

Sexuality encapsulates a wealth of emotions and experience and this makes it hard to grasp as a concept. But the difficulties of understanding and defining it are largely avoided, and sexuality is presented in simplistic terms. Thus, nurses are being asked to incorporate a consideration of the patient's sexuality into nursing care without a basic understanding of what this includes.

There are other reasons why the issue of sexuality is evaded by nurses. First, it is assumed within nursing that, regardless of their age and experience of life, nurses can confidently deal with their patients' sexuality because they have come to terms with their own. This may be an unrealistic expectation. First of all, sexuality is influenced by all manner of experience. It undergoes change and shifts in emphasis throughout life and is a constant source of challenge. Although life experience may help the nurse to cope with sexuality more confidently, it is doubtful whether anyone is ever completely at ease with this aspect of their being.

Second, present-day expectations of nurses ignore the effect of sexuality on the nurse-patient relationship itself, with important implications for the way in which nurses actually work. Clearly the relationship between each nurse and patient will be influenced by both of their personalities and personal histories. In addition, the nature of their interaction may be influenced by the public images or stereotypes of nurses currently available. Moreover, although institutionalisation or the processes of disease may have a profound effect on sexuality, patients nonetheless remain sexual beings. Similarly, nurses do not cease to be human by virtue of being at work. They are not disembodied creatures without any self-awareness. Yet we take it for granted that these same human and self-conscious individuals will be able to cope with the re-markable access they have to the bodies and emotions of their patients—an intimacy generally reserved for, or even prohibited to, the patient's nearest and dearest.

These important factors—the changing nature of individual sexuality and sexuality's all-pervasiveness (for example, the way it can influence work relationships and standards of care) are not widely acknowledged or made acceptable topics of discussion within nurse training. Small wonder then if nurses, struggling alone with the hidden dimensions of the nurse-patient relationship, find it difficult to deal with those elements of the patient's sexuality that nursing *does* recognise to be of legitimate concern.

The purpose of this book is to address these very issues. It is not a manual of the effects of ill health on sexual function but a discussion of sexuality and of the problems that prevent the incorporation of what has been called 'sexual health care' into nursing. It aims to highlight the way in which sexuality is intertwined with nursing (both the process and the institution) and how nurses can be helped to cope with the problems this raises. Much of the content of this book is not 'hard' information as such but arguments and ideas presented with a view to provoking discussion. Formal definitions are avoided, as sexuality seems undefinable in any useful way. Instead, the book develops a picture of what sexuality involves by looking at it from a number of perspectives, such as those found within the social sciences or different accounts of personal experience. The intention is to give nurses a very broad theoretical basis from which to practise, to allow them to weigh up individual patients' needs and respond as each situation demands.

The book is written unashamedly with the nurse in mind as much as the patient. Incorporating the consideration of sexuality into nursing care represents an enormous challenge for any nurse. All too often, nurses are urged to consider the needs of the patient without any parallel consideration of what can feasibly be asked of the nurse or any thought as to how nurses can be supported in their work. This point came out in many of the interviews I conducted with nurses while researching this book. I also draw on my own experience as a nurse and as a patient. As a result, any suggestions I make concerning improvements in nursing practice are limited by what I hope is a realistic understanding of the practical and emotional constraints nurses face.

Explanation of terms

For the sake of simplicity the term 'ill health' denotes not only the presence of disease but also the effects of treatment such as surgery or drugs. It also includes changes in health status (such as injury or decreased mobility) which have to be adjusted to.

Reference is made to both the nursing process and the process of nursing. By *nursing process* I mean of course the method by which nursing care is planned. The *process of nursing* is much more general, referring to the whole endeavour of nursing, including informal and often unacknowledged elements of care such as the use of touch and the interaction between nurse and patient.

When the term 'patient' appears in this book it has been consciously chosen in preference to 'client'. Although 'client' is now in common use it does not, I believe, always reflect the true situation of the person seeking health care. A client is someone using the services of a professional person. To begin with this suggests that a patient as client has some involvement in determining the kind of health care he or she receives. Sadly, this is not always the case. The introduction of the nursing process may be paralleled by a recognition of people's right to be involved in the planning of their care, but for a number of reasons, there remains something of a lag between the overall objectives of nursing and the actual care that is provided.

Second, the term 'client' implies that the relationship between carer and cared for is essentially an equal one. But just as there are well recognised dimensions of power in the doctor-patient relationship, so there is often an imbalance of power between nurses and those they nurse. (Later in the book this power dynamic will be examined in more detail.) For these reasons I think that, in most situations, 'patient' remains a more appropriate term to describe the nurse's subject.

I did not wish to litter the text with references. However, as some of the book is contentious it seemed best to support its arguments with references to other work already published. Moreover, most books represent only one bite of the cherry. It therefore seems important to provide sources of information so that interested readers can build a fuller picture of the subject for themselves, or find alternative interpretations. Where certain information is not drawn upon but may be of interest or help, it is suggested as 'Further Reading' at the end of the appropriate chapter.

2

The nature of sexuality

This section incorporates arguments from disciplines such as psychology, sociology, anthropology and philosophy, to gain as broad as possible a picture of what 'sexuality' should include. The same theme underlies most of these arguments: that sexuality, gender, differences between the sexes, sexual practices and the erotic, are not just biological but largely socially influenced.

What is meant by sexuality?

For any individual, sexuality involves a certain 'self-concept' (which is closely akin to a sense of self-worth); a particular view of the body and its relationship to others; and acceptance to a greater or lesser extent of a specific masculine or feminine gender role, as well as of physical needs which may be sexual or non-sexual, such as the need to be touched. Sexuality refers to more than sexual acts.

Within the nursing literature, sexuality is often portrayed as something totally wholesome and good, 'a voyage into one's own body, mind and spirit which then enriches other dimensions of life', a 'celebration of living' or 'an acknowledgement of different aspects of oneself'. While of course it *can* be all these things, sexuality is not all hearts and flowers, it also has more negative aspects. Sexuality can be the vehicle for the expression of power, dependency, hostility or hatred, as rape, or the sexual abuse of children show us.

Many of the elements of sexuality will be discussed in more

depth later in this chapter. At this stage, however, the fundamental point is summed up by Stone, who says, 'Despite appearances, human sex takes place mostly in the head' (1977:483). Like all things human, sexuality is largely a social phenomenon, meaningful because we endow it with meaning. However, the different meanings given to sexuality, on both a global and personal scale, appear to be endless. This view of sexuality may seem strange. After all, most Western theories of sexuality over the past 100 years (from, for example, Freud, Havelock Ellis, Fromm, Reich, Marcuse or Kinsey) have stated or implied that sexuality is an innate or natural force. It has been assumed that this so-called instinctive, even 'animal' aspect of the human, despite social attempts at control, is so overpowering that it will always express itself. It will become evident either as sexual activity or, indirectly, as perversion or neurosis.

More recently, though, it has been recognised that sexuality is not an innate drive. Nor is sexual development an isolated, inner process. It is shaped throughout life by everyday interactions with others (see Gagnon and Simon 1973). People become sexual just as they become anything else—by picking up cues from their social environment within specific cultural and historical circumstances. Because sexuality is learned through social interaction, sexual meaning is essentially ambiguous. If a woman touches a man in an intimate way while he lies on a couch (for example if she touches his genitals) this *can* be seen as a sexual act on her part. But the same intimate touch can be interpreted as non-sexual if the woman is a doctor conducting a medical examination. Whether this situation is sexually arousing for either party becomes largely dependent on the context and intentions of the parties involved. There has to be a recognition of the sexual nature of this interaction for it to *be* sexual. Plummer (1982) has made precisely this point. To show the way in which sexual meaning may vary he asks which of the following activities can be interpreted as 'sexual':

a child playing with its genitals,
a man kissing another in public,
a woman taking her clothes off in public, or
a mortuary attendant touching a corpse.

Plummer points out that each of these situations *could* be described as sexual by some people—but only in some situations. The context and intentions of the actors are all-important.

Not only is sexuality socially influenced, it can also itself be a powerful social force. It can be used to express inequalities in power, as Groth and others (1977) have shown. Analysing the accounts of both rape survivors and convicted rapists they found most incidents of rape could be identified as the use of sexuality by men to express power or anger, rather than as the outcome of uncontrolled passion.

Sex may represent power in other ways too. In societies where a person needs offspring to achieve power or status, heterosexual intercourse becomes something of a political act. And as Millet (1977) has pointed out, the biological sex into which one is born is significant because of the social implications of being male or female. In most societies, male sex and masculine gender are necessary for the attainment of power or prestige.

Sexuality: public versus private

So far, it has been argued that whether in the form of sex or of gender, sexuality can be used to express socially held values. But however sexuality is represented at the social level, it nonetheless has a personal, possibly very different, meaning for the individual. Where, for example, the social view exists that sex is sinful except as a means to procreation, individuals may still value and enjoy this aspect of their sexuality whether they exercise it in the cause of procreation or not. Whatever the public view, at a *personal* level sex may act as a way of expressing emotions such as love or hostility. Alternatively, it can be used to reassure self-identity. It may also be the means by which individuals experience themselves as part of a much wider scheme of things, that is, as part of a cosmic order. Sexual experience holds different meanings for different people. While this may sound an obvious point, it is central to an understanding not only of the relationship between public and private understandings of sexuality but also of the differences between male and female sexuality.

Male and female sexuality

If sexuality is largely shaped by social influences rather than biology, why do we see clear differences between male and female sexual behaviour? In Western culture men are assumed to be more sexually aggressive than women. It is thought that they will 'by nature' take the initiative in sex as in other spheres of life. They are supposedly quick to be sexually aroused and satisfied. They are automatically credited with a strong libido (or sex drive), so 'needing' sex more frequently than women. Conversely women are thought to be sexually passive. Because of a weak libido, they are more responsive than assertive. They are understood to be prone to problems with either sexual arousal or climax. Surely, if sexuality were merely a social phenomenon we could not draw such a clear distinction between male and female sexual behaviour?

To answer this question we first have to be sure that these differences between men and women actually exist, and are not just stereotypes we have come to accept unquestioningly. Women's libido, for example, has been variously described in different eras both as totally insatiable and as non-existent (see Stone *ibid*; McLaren 1984). Today, female sexuality is regarded as a rather insipid variation on male sexuality. This view, like its predecessors, represents just one facet of a more general, contemporary understanding of women, men and the relationship between them. Second, researchers such as Hite (1977, 1981) have shown that there is considerable variation within both male and female sexuality, of which homosexuality is one example. Third, if any differences in sexual behaviour do exist between the sexes, there is very little at the biological level to explain them. In fact, as the sexologists Masters and Johnson have demonstrated, there are great physiological similarities between men and women. The clitoris, for example, is not, as has been suggested, an inferior version of the penis. Both are supplied with a similar network of veins and nerves and each is potentially as sensitive to stimulation as the other. This is not surprising as, developmentally, both are derived from the same embryonic structure, the undifferentiated genital tubercle.

Apparent differences between male and female sexual behaviour therefore do not, by and large, come about as the result of different biology. Instead, where differences exist they have to be seen predominantly as the outcome of the social implications of being either a man or a woman. Sexual behaviour, even solitary masturbation, occurs in a social context and is shaped more by social expectations of men and women (that is, gender) than by anatomy and physiology. This becomes clear if we take a specific example of the link between sexual behaviour and gender role.

Many men use sexuality to demonstrate social dominance. Rape is the extreme example of this. In other less violent contexts doubts about masculinity can be assuaged by a 'successful' sexual encounter—success being measured in terms of conquest as opposed to the giving of pleasure to a sexual partner. However, male sexuality is something of a paradox, acting as a vehicle for both domination and dependency. In Western culture, men are generally denied ways of expressing dependency and need other than through sexuality, or more precisely, genital sex. Men appear to seek sex for its own sake more often than women but this may be because it allows them to give and receive tenderness in a way that would otherwise be seen as unmanly.

Erotic sex

So far, we have been principally considering the erotic aspect of sexuality, or erotic sex. 'Erotic' is a deceptive work, concealing a complex range of meanings and feelings. People may become sexually excited by quite different stimuli. An individual may be aroused by a certain experience on one occasion but not on another. This suggest that *desire*, one element of eroticism, has little basis in biology (Rickford 1983). Admittedly, erotic sex has a biological component in that sex usually involves some form of outward physicality, and erotic stimuli may produce inner physiological responses such as the changes demonstrated by Masters and Johnson (see pp. 10–13). However, this is not the end of the matter. What happens in bed (or elsewhere) is largely determined by what happens out of it. Angela Carter puts it concisely:

'We do not go to bed in simple pairs; even if we choose not to refer to them, we still drag there with us the cultural impedimenta of our social class, our parents' lives, our bank balances, our sexual and emotional expectations, our whole biographies—all the bits and pieces of our unique existences. (1982:9)

Erotic sex has economic and social implications. How much sex we have and with whom can lead to us being categorised as, for example, 'slut', as if this kind of description can in some way totally define us. And as Root (1984) points out, welfare and housing policy, law, employment and so on may benefit some types of sexual relationships more than others. For example, a woman who lives alone but has a long-term heterosexual relationship has a different entitlement to Social Security than a woman who lives with her male lover. In some types of employment a married man will be given preference for a job over an unmarried man because having a wife supposedly makes him more reliable. Conversely, an unmarried woman without children is often given preference over a married woman with children (or even a woman of childbearing age), as it is assumed that her domestic commitments will interfere with her work.

The supposed overpowering, innate force of sexuality can be seen to lose much of its 'compulsion' in the face of the economic. Ortner and Whitehead (1981) point out that it is only necessary to remember that Imperial China never seemed to lack recruits to the Palace staff of eunuchs (who would apply for work bringing their genitals with them in a jar) to be reminded of the extent to which social and economic considerations can override those of the libido.

Erotic sex covers a multitude of acts and desires. It includes non-penetrative, non-genital, homosexual, heterosexual, bi-sexual and group sex, and masturbation. The term 'sex' used in this context therefore refers to anything that has erotic meaning for the individual. (The other use of the term is discussed under the heading 'Biological sex'.)

Masters and Johnson have looked at what happens physiologically during erotic sex. Because their findings have gone a long way towards challenging many assumptions about sexuality, and as their work often provides the basis for psychosexual therapy, it is worth looking at in some detail here. However, this is only one model of sexual response. In contrast to their four phases of response, for example, Kaplan (1974) has identified a bi-phasic cycle of response. Her model is not as well known or as accepted as Masters' and Johnson's but its very existence emphasises that sexual response can be interpreted in different ways—even at the physiological level.

Masters and Johnson

As a result of empirical studies, Masters and Johnson claim that

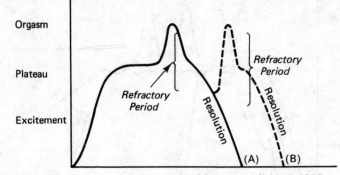

Figure 1   *The male sexual response cycle (Masters and Johnson 1966).*

the physiological response of both men and women to sexual stimulation can be divided into four stages: the phases of excitement, plateau, orgasm and resolution. The excitement phase is characterised by physiological changes such as widespread vaso-congestion, which occurs as a response to mental or physical sexual stimulation. If this stimulation continues, the first phase gives way to a second, the plateau phase, in which sexual tension is increased to the level at which orgasm becomes possible. The orgasmic phase is that in which involuntary climax occurs and it is here that potential differences between the sexes begin to emerge. Among men there is relatively little variation in terms of the intensity of the climax, while there is great variation in both the intensity and duration of female orgasm. Further differences emerge in the fourth stage. For men the duration of the resolution phase is partially fixed by what is known as the 'refractory period' or the time during which renewed sexual stimulation will have little physiological effect. A second erection will not be possible immediately after orgasm. This refractory period varies with age, generally increasing in later years. It will either be followed by resolution and the dissipation of any remaining sexual tension (see 'A' in Figure 1) or, in the presence of further stimulation, may be followed by a repeat of the phases of plateau and orgasm, followed by a further refractory period and then resolution (see 'B' in Figure 1). In comparison women have the potential for an infinite variety of response patterns. For example, as they have no refractory period they *can* experience multiple orgasms—provided there is effective stimulation. ('A', 'B', and 'C' in Figure 2 represent

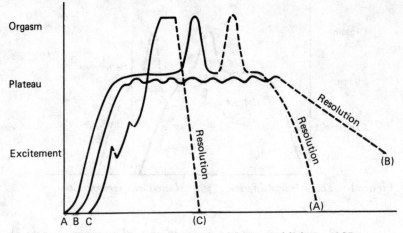

Figure 2   *The female sexual response cycle* (*Masters and Johnson 1966*).

simplifications of just some of the response patterns that Masters and Johnson observed.)

Despite these differences, it is the *similarities* between male and female response at the level of anatomy and physiology that Masters and Johnson wish to emphasise (1966:8). We must suspect that something other than biology is at work when we see different forms of sexuality emerging (even at simply the erotic level) between women and men. However, Masters and Johnson tell only part of the story. Despite their biological potential for multiple orgasm, many women never experience a single climax—for essentially social reasons, and the single, isolated climax of the male remains generally the ideal pattern of events for both men and women. In the popular understanding of male and female sexual response, the differences that exist at a biological level, that is, the different potentials for orgasm, are generally ignored, while the non-biological differences—for example, women's supposedly weaker sexual response—are emphasised.

The contribution made by Masters and Johnson to the understanding of human sexuality is undeniably valuable in a number of respects. Not only have they demonstrated the similarities between male and female sexual response and provided a general understanding of the physiology involved, but they have also helped to debunk a number of myths. Their work has shown that the physical expression of sexuality does not lose its importance for the elderly, as is often assumed. They have demonstrated that masturbation, instead of being a harmful and depraved act of self-abuse, is important for teaching individuals about their own mode of sexual response and their own particular sexual needs. Further-more, Masters and Johnson have disproved Freud's view of female sexuality which saw only the woman who experienced 'vaginal orgasm' (orgasm resulting from vaginal penetration) as sexually mature. Instead they have shown the centrality of the clitoris in most orgasmic experience, whether or not it is associated with penetration of the vagina, and so paved the way towards a better understanding of female sexuality. And Masters and Johnson deserve credit for providing the basis for a form of sex therapy which has been tremendously helpful for many people. But despite the positive aspects of their work, it is important for at least two reasons that their contribution should not be seized upon as the essence of any understanding of erotic sexuality.

Sexual excitement in the laboratory

First, Masters and Johnson (and other sexologists, such as Kinsey) have placed enormous emphasis on the orgasm. Largely as a re-sult of the Masters and Johnson model of the four stages of sexual response, erotic sexuality in the West has been 'framed' as goal-oriented, to the extent that sexual fulfilment has become entirely synonymous with orgasm. It should be remembered though that this model was developed from clinical observation of physio-logical response to sexual excitement in the laboratory. Of course most people do not live in laboratory conditions. While I do not dispute many of Masters' and Johnson's conclusions, as they themselves acknowledge, their research sample was not represent-ative of the general American public from which it was drawn. It was untypical not only because people were being asked to make love in a highly unusual context, but also because many volun-teers came from the local academic community. Subjects were also unrepresentative because they usually experienced orgasm—even in laboratory conditions. It is also possible that the very nature and context of the study influenced the volunteers' be-haviour so that, for example, orgasm became a focus in a way it might not have otherwise.

Data resulting from the observation of this research group was subsequently formalised so that Masters' and Johnson's findings are presented to us as a neat pattern of four stages. They themselves take pains to stress that this is a simplification, but it is the formal model of four stages that has come to determine many people's expectations of what they should experience. As a result, sexual excitement is widely understood to move in linear progression according to a set pattern, even if the intensity and duration of the experiences are understood to vary. This pattern is not always evident in real life. Actual sexual experience may not correspond to the 'A', 'B', 'C' and 'D' stages of the Masters and Johnson model, let alone conform to their sequential ordering. For example, ejaculation can happen without erection and *vice versa* (Kaplan *ibid*). Nor does sex have to follow the famous four stages to be pleasurable or satisfying.

Second, Masters' and Johnson's classic work is based on a drive theory of sexuality in which the biological nature of sexual motivation is seen to be as compelling as the need for food and drink. It fails to do justice to the *meaning* that sexual acts hold for individuals or their emotional associations. Masters and Johnson emphasise the mutual enjoyment of sexual activity as the basis of marital happiness but this sexual activity appears quite detached from whatever else is going on in the marriage. The couple in therapy are encouraged to practise 'good sex' with the aim of maintaining their marriage and family but without looking at the overall marital relationship or the pressures from within or outside the family that may influence sexual interaction (Segal 1983). Recent work by Masters takes a different stance but it is this earlier approach which informs many people's understanding of sexuality.

Masters and Johnson have given us a wealth of information about the physiology of sexual response. And there is no doubt that poor theoretical knowledge of anatomy and physiology can, in part, be the cause of an unsatisfying sexual relationship. But reading a text book will not necessarily inform anyone of the particular needs of a specific partner. Moreover, the wish to learn what gives pleasure to a lover most probably correlates with the socially determined dynamic of the relationship. A male/female relationship is often a more or less equal one—with the man more and the woman less equal! Significantly, social inequality can provide one of the strongest erotic charges—at least for those weighing in with greater shares of power. As Kissinger is quoted as saying, 'Power is the ultimate aphrodisiac'.

Biological sex

Besides referring to the erotic, the term 'sex' has a further meaning—the anatomically defined characteristics of maleness or femaleness. Biological sex covers a number of sub-categories. Dewhurst (1981) distinguishes five: chromosomal sex, gonadal sex, sex of internal and external genitalia and sex of rearing (or gender). I would argue there are essentially only four: gender does not belong under this heading as it is not biological.

In biological sex, chromosomes determine maleness or femaleness (that is, chromosomal sex), the female having two X sex chromosomes and the male one X and one Y. The pattern of an individual's chromosomes provides their chromosomal sex and is unchangeable. Normally testes will develop in the early embryo if a Y chromosome is present. Ovaries develop if the Y chromosome is absent and there are at least two X chromosomes. Presence of either ovary or testis is known as gonadal or primary sex. Once testes are present the individual will develop male genitals. However, without the formation of testes (or if the gonads should be removed from the embryo before gonadal differentiation takes place) female genital organs will develop irrespective of chromosomal sex and regardless of whether ovaries are present or not. Interestingly, some have used this sequence of development to claim that the female is the 'asexual' norm (Dewhurst: *ibid*), while others have seen the development of male gonadal sex as a glorious 'fight to be male' (for example, Goldwyn 1979). These descriptions are misleading and are often used to imply that there are biological origins for cultural characteristics such as aggression in men.

The developing fetus has the potential for both female (Müllerian) and male (Wolffian) internal reproductive systems; development of one or other system depends in part on the presence or absence of high androgen and testosterone levels, but both sexes have some levels of both male and female hormones. Embryologically, the external genital organs are the last to develop and it is not all that uncommon for them to be left unfinished. It is the appearance of these organs (which can sometimes be misleading) that will generally decide the gender to which the child will be expected to conform.

Gender: masculinity and femininity

Just as sexuality can be looked at from both social and individual perspectives, so gender also has two different aspects, the public and the private. *Gender role* is the public aspect of gender, referring to attitudes, characteristics, behaviour and even jobs which are, within a particular culture, thought to accompany biological maleness or femaleness. It includes everything a person publicly says or does to demonstrate the degree to which they fit the cultural view of masculinity or femininity. *Gender identity* is the private or inner experience of gender. It describes an individual's awareness of gender, or personal definitions of masculinity or femininity which may not always correspond with cultural gender roles.

Unfortunately, gender is an area in which the biological and the social are frequently confused. For example, terms such as 'female' and 'feminine' are often used interchangeably, although they actually mean quite different things. While 'female' refers to chromosomal (i.e. biological) sex, 'femininity' refers to socially-defined characteristics that are attributed to women (i.e. gender). Most cultures consider that there is a natural link between male or female anatomy and what counts as masculine or feminine behaviour; gender *appears* to be the outcome of sexual difference. In reality, however, the way in which behavioural characteristics are allotted to men or women is a social process, not a natural one. As Strathern (1976) has pointed out, gender is a set of *ideas*, which underlie the way a society builds certain stereotypes and roles.

Links between gender and health have helped to confuse gender and biology. Clearly some illnesses occur more often among one sex than the other. Men are more likely to suffer heart disease than women (although this trend is shifting) and women are more prone to mental disorders than men. It is important though to understand that these problems are not sex-linked— they are not genetically determined—but are linked to the social and cultural meanings attached to being either male or female, in other words, to gender.

Women are thought to be more prone to psychiatric morbidity than men, not because they experience more life events, but because they experience more events of an undesirable nature as a result of their lower socio-economic state. Women are more likely to have less income and lower occupational status then men, even if they are in similar jobs. It is these sorts of differences in the *social* environment, rather than any constitutional differences between women and men that appear to lead to higher rates of mental ill health among women (Jenkins and Clare 1985). Gove (1984) has shown that traditionally, male roles are more highly structured than female ones, and this is related to relatively good mental health. In contrast, the nurturant roles such as child care which are usually occupied by women are not clearly defined. They do not, for instance, end neatly at five o'clock. These roles impose a specific kind of strain which limits women's ability to accept a sick role, and are ultimately associated with poor mental health (see also Roberts 1985).

Gender roles promote what is known as the 'sexual division of labour', in which each sex becomes associated with tasks, such as breadwinning or housekeeping, according to cultural concepts of the behaviour appropriate for men and women. This comes to be accepted as the *natural* outcome of sex differences. In Western culture the biological adaptation of the female for childbirth and feeding of the very young has come to be accepted as an argument for women's *long-term* involvement with children and fitness for nurturing roles in general. Men, because of their role as breadwinner, are seen to have become 'naturally' more aggressive than women in order to be able to compete for resources in the outside world. These behavioural differences between the sexes are assumed to be genetic in origin and, by implication, not only right and proper but also unchangeable.

But it can also be argued that while men and women are specialised for different reproductive roles, and while there is an undeniable genetic basis to some of the physical differences between the sexes, this does not need to determine individual behaviour. Instead, there is a continuous interplay between an individual and his or her social environment. Strength, for example, may depend partly on muscular endowment but also partly on training. As a rule, women have less muscle than men, but some women are stronger than some men. The way in which genetic differences between the sexes (such as muscle size) are expressed, for example, as notable differences in strength, will depend on environmental and social factors, including the way in which available food is distributed or whether girls are given encouragement and facilities for sport from an early age (Lieven 1981).

The social basis of gender can be seen in cross-cultural variations in concepts of masculinity or femininity. Among some peoples, gender is not strongly emphasised. The Arapesh of New Guinea, for instance, see both men and women as gentle and nurturing, while the Mundugumou of New Guinea regard both sexes as equally assertive and independent. Others perceive marked gender distinctions. The Tcambuli—also of New Guinea—regard women as aggressive while men are caring and more suited for domestic tasks, turning Western stereotypes inside out (Oakley 1972). In some cultures, gender concepts do not directly correspond with any distinctions drawn between men and women. Shore (1981), studying gender and sexuality in Samoa, found that all men were understood to have some feminine characteristics and all women some masculine ones. Moreover, some men were recognised as having more developed female elements in their personality than most, to the extent that they were given a special status—a third gender category beyond 'masculine' or 'feminine'.

The social basis of gender can also be observed in Western culture. Money and Ehrhardt (1972), for example, describe case histories of boys who had anatomical abnormalities of the genitals which led to them being raised as girls. In childhood these boys adopted typically feminine patterns of behaviour and posture and took on a typically feminine gender role. Unfortunately, what happened to them in later life has not been studied. The available evidence, however, suggests that what was important in deciding gender identity was not their biological sex but the way in which they were raised (see also Singleton 1986).

How is gender identity formed, if it is not innate? Gender socialisation can be seen to begin at birth, or rather from the moment when a child's genitalia are interpreted as either male or female. From this time on, concepts of gender are highly influential in determining the child's upbringing, moulding, for example, dress, the degree of attention and mental stimulation he or she will receive, expectations of play behaviour and—later on—career choice, hobbies, etc. The forms of influence are many. Child-rearing practices play an important role. So does peer group pressure. There are also other, less tangible but powerful influences ranging from the advertising industry to the medical profession (see pp. 21–24).

There are several ways of understanding the development of masculine or feminine identity. Some explanations are more credible than others, and none fully explains the way in which gender is learned. Each argument, though, contributes something to our understanding of the process.

One approach stems from a Freudian psychoanalytical understanding of development and emphasises anatomical differences as a basis for difference in masculine or feminine identity. 'Absence' of the penis, for example, supposedly leads to 'penis envy' among women. But as de Beauvoir says (1975), *if* women do envy men anything, it is most likely to be the almost exclusive hold on power that they have (which may be symbolised by the penis) rather than the penis itself.

Social learning theory sees masculine and feminine identity as resulting from conditions in the social environment which help shape personality. Masculinity and femininity represent certain social values which are learned by children and taken as their own. The problem with this view is that it often sees conformity to gender stereotypes as development *per se* and fails to recognise that masculinity and femininity are not simple concepts automatically and cumulatively acquired with age.

A third, more developmental theory takes into account the way that masculine or feminine identities represent *changing* ways of interpreting differences between the sexes; that gender is not a stable phenomenon which remains on a fixed course of development throughout life. Instead, this third approach more convincingly explains why individuals do not always conform to prevailing gender stereotypes and why, in our culture for example, we have witnessed the relatively recent trends of women entering the building trades and men going into nursing. The capacity for change implied by this view of gender development has an important meaning for those whose gender role and gender identity are challenged by ill health. The undermining of a person's sense of masculinity or femininity can be demoralising and depressing. It is perhaps one of the most fundamental, if subtle, ways in which sexuality can be affected by illness. An important element of nursing care, therefore, has to be to help the patient understand the nature of gender identity and come to terms with change. This involves providing information which allows patients to see that the gender role they take as a model and strive to maintain is not the only role open to them.

The relationship between gender and sexuality

What is the relationship between gender and sexuality? Both are partly social and partly personal constructs, yet though inter-related, they are not synonymous. McKeighen (1978) shows something of the intertwined nature of the relationship. She describes how gender identity begins at birth with the assignment of sex according to external genitalia and becomes well established by the age of two. Then (along with other aspects of identity such as age or culture) it begins to influence general mannerisms, dress, conduct, play preference, content of dreams, daydreams, fantasies and erotic practices. Gender identity would thus appear to have an important influence on erotic sexuality.

Conversely, almost the opposite can happen. Sexuality, or its erotic aspect, can help support gender identity (Person 1980). In Western culture, genital sexuality is often a prominent feature of gender identity and especially important in bolstering up masculine identity. A man suffering from impotence, for example, feels that not only his sexuality but his masculinity is threatened by his inability to get an erection. Strangely, it seems that femininity is not threatened to the same extent by the ups and downs of a woman's sex life. This seems to be partly because for women in our culture, gender identity can be strengthened by other means, such as a feminine appearance or the carrying out of accepted feminine roles, for example, by clothes and cosmetics, or through domesticity.

There is no inevitable link between gender socialisation and sexual behaviour: that is, gender identity does not necessarily determine sexual practice. For instance, if women are socially passive (if, for example, they allow men to make most of their decisions for them) it does not follow that they will be passive in bed. To assume this is to overlook the distinction between gender and eroticism (Barrett 1980). The observations of sexologists suggest that a wide range of sexual behaviour exists that is inconsistent with ascribed gender roles. The lack of any automatic link between erotic behaviour and gender identity is also underlined in the instance of homosexuality. One of the oldest myths about homosexuality is that it is the outcome of some sort of gender imbalance. While each of us has masculine and feminine elements, the possession of 'too much' masculinity by women or 'too much' femininity by men has been thought to 'cause' homosexuality.

This view is now strongly contested. It overlooks, for example, the fact that masculine identity remains important to many men who are homosexual. Indeed, according to Brake (1982), masculinity is given a privileged status in both heterosexual and homosexual worlds. Brandes, an anthropologist, studied the residents of an Andalusian town (1981). He found male homosexuality an accepted practice, carrying no social stigma *provided* a man consistently took what was understood as a masculine role. This meant being the partner who initiated sex and, if penetration was involved, being the penetrator and not the penetrated. Receptiveness to penetration was regarded as analogous to feminine behaviour and as such, shameful. Revelation of passivity was therefore dreaded.

Thus, masculinity may be an important consideration for many gay men. Similarly femininity may be central to a lesbian's identity. The categorisation of 'active' and 'passive' partners however has to be seen as an aspect of a specific form of sexuality which can be found among both some homosexuals and some heterosexuals. It should not be seen as yet another stereotype of homosexuality. The categories of 'butch' and 'femme' for instance—so often thought to be a central dynamic of lesbianism—do not actually describe contemporary Western lesbian relationships.

To summarise, the same (social) factors that influence the construction of gender categories such as masculinity or femininity also have *some* effect on the adoption of 'appropriate' erotic behaviour and other aspects of sexuality. It cannot be said that there is *no* link between gender and sexuality. However there is no *inevitable* link between the two. Sexuality can be interpreted by the individual according to his or her needs (if with difficulty) and this potential freedom of interpretation, as suggested earlier, has important implications for nursing care.

The social construction of gender and sexuality

Before ending this section we should consider the ways in which gender and sexuality are socially constructed. In other words, how our emotions, desires and relationships are to a large extent shaped by the society and culture in which we live. The forms of influence are many. An implicit definition of 'appropriate' sexual behaviour can be found within DHSS rulings. The medical profession can also play a powerful part in the way we understand sexuality and gender. Scully and Bart (1978) have shown how gynaecologists (generally men) have become official specialists, not only of female reproductive pathology, but also of women as a whole. They are often in the privileged position of defining 'normal sexuality' and 'normal femininity'. The social sciences are another sphere of influence. According to Macintyre (1976), for instance, sociologists by and large fail to look at what they call 'normal' reproduction—namely the bearing of children within marriage. It is assumed that this is the normal way to do things, and does not require investigation. Instead research has largely concentrated on so-called 'abnormal' behaviour—for example, on why married women might want abortions or, conversely, why unmarried women might wish to become mothers. By their very definitions, by choosing to concentrate on some forms of behaviour and ignoring others, sociologists play their part in building a particular understanding of sexuality. These are brief examples of ways in which gender and sexuality can be socially constructed. Before leaving the subject I would like to provide one further example in more detail.

Advertisements and sexuality

The advertising industry creates desire in order to sell products. As part of this process it frequently invents its own images of what it is to be a man or a woman. It may also promote or exaggerate existing images.

In contemporary advertisements women are usually portrayed either as pleasant looking if sexually neutral wives and mothers or as glamorous and ever available sex-objects. The treatment of men has been quite different until very recently. Men in adverts are usually doing something or possessing something; actively making their way in the world rather than awaiting inspection and approval. They may be handsome, but just as often have features which suggest 'character' or weathering by experience. This aspect is absent from most images of women; there is no obvious suggestion that women have been engaged in life's rich tapestry.

The asymmetry of masculine and feminine stereotypes is not just created by the media. What is significant, however, is that the media sharpen what is seen as masculine or feminine and provide the stereotype with visibility and greater validity. Media images become highly influential in developing individual men's and women's perceptions of masculinity and femininity.

Reuhl (1983) shows how the commercial construction of certain images of women becomes an unquestioned part of modern consumerism. The image of a naked woman may be used to sell something quite unrelated to nakedness or to women—like a fork-lift truck! Advertisements demand at some level that we make some connection between the product and the image used to sell it, but in reality the link is often nonsensical. The real absurdity of using a woman's body to state something about the majority of products is demonstrated by a spoof advertisement published by *Time Out*. A man, dressed in a pair of briefs and smoking a pipe, reclines with legs sprawled on the bonnet of a car. According to the 'logic' of advertising, there should be some connection between the image of this half-naked man and the qualities of the car which will compel people to buy it. But because of the reversal of the stereotype we can see the ridiculous nature of the pose and the extremely tenuous link between the image being promoted and the product.

In advertisements, women's bodies are often used in a way that suggests their sexual availability rather than representing an active female sexuality. Women's breasts have come to represent male rather than female sexuality. When they appear in advertisements it is generally to sell products to men. Interestingly, men's bodies are appearing more often in adverts but they are used in a very different way. Despite its increased display and commercialisation, the male form remains less of an object than the female body. It is somehow still active and possessing despite being unclothed. This is because it is presented with a male rather than a female audience in mind. This trend is in part a response to the expanding 'gay' market. It also represents a shift in the way men in general are being prompted to view themselves as more body-conscious. But the underlying concept of masculinity remains more or less unchanged: images of hardness—whether of hard muscles or symbols for hard penises—are still used to signify masculinity/male sexuality and continue to work against any association between men and softness or tenderness. The soft penis is just not considered capable of shifting merchandise!

Generally speaking, most analyses of the construction of gender and sexuality have been concerned with images of women and femininity. Craik (1979), for example, has shown how advertisements construct a sense of the feminine as something mysterious and unknowable. She gives the example of a Guy Laroche advert for perfume. The slogan reads: 'Woman is an island. Fidgi is her perfume'. Now just what does this mean? Significantly it is not *a* woman who is an island (which carries a presumably undesirable message of isolation), but *Woman*—suggesting an abstract, feminine essence which is mysterious and yet at the same time we can all be expected to agree on its nature. The minimal use of words endorses the suggestion; the fewer the words, the greater the mystery. Furthermore, failure to understand the nature of the mystery carries the implication that we are not truly feminine (or masculine) ourselves. This example shows how advertisers do not represent any form of reality, instead creating blank sheets on which to draw masculinity or femininity in whichever way is best calculated to sell their products. They create forms of gender that most suit their interests. What should also be considered are the adverse effects of this sort of strategy.

Advertisements depict, and to a large extent create, a valuation in Western culture of a slim female body and a hard male one. We have already seen how media images work against any association between men and tenderness. The value placed on slimness in women means that those who do not conform to the ideal often feel 'too big', that they occupy too much space. They feel their body alone proclaims to the world that they are inadequate in some way as it appears they cannot control their appetites (Coward 1984). The media in general have been in the forefront of making image or appearance more important than anything else and of making conformity to the norm the basis of being desirable. Orbach has made this point in saying that a woman's body has been turned into a commodity for use in the pursuit of happiness (1982). Received wisdom says that slimness can be equated with both health and happiness, but this is a dubious claim. For many women, fatness can become a way of rejecting the demand to conform to a packaged identity—if at the risk of their health.

This shows once again how important it is for nurses to have a thorough understanding of gender as a social construct (and therefore not an inevitability) in order to help their patients challenge gender roles which may pose some threat to their physical or emotional health.

Sexual health and sexual health care

It is widely acknowledged that the increasing emphasis on sexuality within nursing is in order to promote sexual health. However, just as sexuality is impossible to define neatly, so too are 'sexual health' and 'sexual health care'.

A report from the World Heath Organisation (WHO) describes sexual health as the capacity to enjoy and control sexual and reproductive behaviour according to social and personal ethics. Furthermore, there should be an absence of disease which affects sexual or reproductive function. There should also be freedom from shame, guilt or misconceptions which might mar sexual relationships (Mace and others 1974). By this definition, sexual health is only concerned with reproduction and the erotic aspects of sexuality. A subsequent WHO report, however, recognised that the purpose of sexual health care should be 'the enhancement of life and personal relationships' (WHO 1975:7). It also acknowledged the difficulties of finding a universally acceptable definition of sexuality which could describe the totality of human sexuality. Nonetheless it attempted to make a move in this direction by suggesting sexual health to be 'the integration of the somatic, emotional, intellectual and social aspects of sexual being in ways that are positively enriching and that enhance personality, communication and love' (ibid:6). This definition undoubtedly gives a better indication of the breadth of sexual health concerns than earlier attempts, but is unfortunately associated with two major problems. First, many writers on sexuality simply 'lift' this definition without referring to the qualifying remarks of its originators; the definition is therefore presented as if it is entirely adequate. Second, the definition is so general that it is difficult to apply. Conversely, being more specific carries the risk that definitions are interpreted too narrowly and create rigid ideas of what constitutes sexual health instead of providing basic guidelines. Maddock (1975), for example, has defined sexual health as having four components:

1. the ability to make mature judgements about personal sexual behaviour in line with one's values and beliefs;
2. the ability to take part in interpersonal relationships with both sexes and in relationships that involve commitment or love;
3. a sense of congruence between having the body of a man or

woman and correspondingly masculine or feminine psychosexual and gender identities;
4. the capacity to respond to erotic stimulation in a way that
makes sexual activity a positive experience.

One problem with this composite definition is that it implies
sexual health is the sum total of all its components. Yet it is quite
possible to be sexually healthy without engaging in erotic sex; for
some people the choice of celibacy represents a mature judgement
about personal sexual behaviour in line with their values and
beliefs. Therefore, as Woods points out about definitions of sexual
health:

> 'As with definitions of general health, these must be applied
> liberally so that lack of a single component is not cause for
> labelling a patient "unhealthy". It is important to keep in mind
> that sexual health is a relative matter; even the most disabled
> person can then be considered sexually healthy.'(1984:86)

The third component of Maddock's definition raises a different
problem. It is dangerous ground to suggest that sexual health
necessarily means that if you have the body of a man, for instance,
your behaviour must be that expected of men by society—that
sexual health entails conforming to gender-role expectations. As
Webb has said, people should not be placed in one or other of the
two categories of masculine or feminine. Nor should they be allocated to a point on a line running between the two opposites of
masculinity or femininity. Whatever their biological sex, people
should have the freedom to behave as they wish in terms of gender
or sexual practice. She points out that the only necessary limit to
this is that the freedom of one person should not harm another
(1985a).

To assume that a congruence between biological sex and
gender-role conformity is necessary for sexual health is to ignore
the way in which society's expectations of behaviour are formed.
Remembering the different influences on ideas of gender, can it
really be that sexual health involves, for example, dancing to the
tune of the DHSS? Surely not.

If nurses are to help patients express their sexuality, as they are
now being urged to do, they should be able to see the arbitrariness
of social norms and expectations. In the provision of sexual health
care they must be prepared to help patients understand their per-

sonal sexual identity and, where appropriate, help them to challenge those aspects of gender role they find oppressive. This is clearly very important for those whose sexual identity is undermined by ill health. However, if sexual health is about coming to terms with different aspects of one's sexuality, together with the freedom to express sexuality, then it is of concern to the vast majority of the population, and may therefore become an issue for the nurse in any area of work. It has to be said that at the moment, nursing practice tends unquestioningly to reinforce gender-role. This is the outcome of a number of problems at both theoretical and practical levels and these will be examined later in the book. Prior to this, Chapters 2 and 3 will look more specifically at what should be encompassed by any reference to the *patient's* sexuality and how sexuality may be affected by ill health. These chapters also demonstrate the breadth of issues involved within the concept of sexual health.

Further reading

Weeks J. (1986). *Sexuality*. Chichester: Ellis Horwood.

3

Non-erotic sexuality in sickness and in health

Introduction

This chapter will look at the non-erotic ways in which the body is experienced in health and illness, exploring the phenomena of self-concept, body-image, spatial relations, body boundary and touch, and making use of research from the social sciences which is usually excluded from nurse education. This may be unfamiliar ground for some nurses, but it is nonetheless highly relevant. Understanding the many ways in which experience of the body can influence self-concept is important for realising what it means for one's body to be threatened by illness or hospitalisation.

Body and space

The body has symbolic as well as biological functions, and symbolic meanings derived from the body's basic processes vary from culture to culture. In many ways, as Merleau-Ponty (1962) has pointed out, our body provides the basis for understanding our personal world.

In Western culture, the body is viewed from a number of different perspectives. Artistic conventions through the ages have given us a range of perceptions of the human body, the images of each era providing indications of what were thought to be fundamental features of being human, including, of course, ideas about masculinity and femininity (MacRae 1975). Our contemporary portrayal of the body provides another new perspective, but which is again linked to wider social issues (see, for example, the earlier discussion of the role of advertising, pp. 22–24).

The body drawn by science or medicine is very different. For medicine the body becomes a number of static images: cross-sectional diagrams, X-rays or graphs of the body's various physiological cycles.

Quite distinct from these representations are our own personal images and experiences. This is the body—our body—that ingests, excretes, has sensation, experiences sexual arousal and so on. Finally, there are the bodies of others as we see them, quite separate from ourselves and linked only on occasion—for example, through sexual intercourse.

Spatial relationships

Our feelings about space and the values we attach to it have been thought to come principally from our body form (MacRae *ibid*). The human body is basically symmetrical and generally thought of as being upright (although it is more often slouched, twisted, recumbent, etc.). From this upright orientation come our categories of direction, such as up, down, right, left, before and behind, together with the values we attach to them. What is above comes to be seen as superior, for example, 'mind over matter'. The body acts as a guide through which the individual organises spatial experience.

The way in which the body is experienced varies historically, cross-culturally and even within one society (for example, according to class and gender). In the contemporary West we generally experience ourselves as isolated beings, with a mind separate from the material body. This view dates from the time of the philosopher Descartes, who in the seventeenth century equated individual identity with the mind, in his famous saying '*Cogito ergo sum*' ('I think therefore I am'). Other philosophies make little distinction between mind and body. There may also be less emphasis on the individual as a separate entity. In Hindu thought, a continuous flow of 'essences' is recognised between all humans. The predominant Eastern world view is an organic one, in which all things known through the senses are interrelated and represent different aspects of the same ultimate reality.

A similar perspective could be found in medieval Europe, when space did not have the same geometrical characteristics it has for us now. There was, for example, little sense of being differentiated from the outside world at the level of the individual body-boundary. People instead seemed to be aware of a connection between themselves and other humans as well as with other animals, plants, minerals, and the heavenly bodies. This connectedness was apparently experienced as we might experience our internal organs today—precise location being less important than the role we understand them to play in our existence (Jones 1983).

In the West today, everyday distinctions between the symbolic and real, inner and outer, subjective and objective are being radically challenged by work in the field of quantum physics. The exploration of the atomic and subatomic worlds in the present century has demonstrated the limitations of classical scientific ideas and now some of the most basic concepts of science are having to be reconsidered. The new concepts of matter, space and time, while totally different from recent Western ideas, are in many respects similar to those of many mystics. Both ways of thought emphasise the interrelation of all phenomena and the idea of a universe as an inseparable whole, the constituents of which are fluid and ever-changing (Capra 1983). Not only is the world now seen as a system of inseparable and interacting components, but the observer is understood as an integral part of this system. There is therefore no clear distinction between self and other, subject and object. As yet these ideas have not affected the way in which the majority of Westerners understand or experience themselves in the world. Our everyday life remains largely influenced by previous philosophies, predominantly those arising from traditional Western science, although holistic approaches within nursing and medicine, for example, are heralding change.

There is no inevitable pattern of spatial relations; our understanding of experience of space is more psychological and social than physical (Jones *ibid*). Just as perception is governed by what we expect to see, so our experience of space is largely determined by our expectations. And these expectations are, to a large extent, socially formed.

This is an important point for nurses. It helps to clarify how the personal space they may infringe in the course of their work may be differently experienced by different people according, for example, to varying family attitudes or cultural expectations. The next part of the chapter examines this aspect more fully.

Proxemics, or cultural space

Hall (1966) has described the ways in which people of different cultures experience space. He suggests there is a general failure to grasp the many elements that contribute towards a human sense of space and that this is due in part to the mistaken notion that the human body begins and ends with the skin. Among middle-class Americans, he has identified a series of zones extending around the body, into which entry by others is governed by certain social conventions. Closest to the body is an *intimate zone*, usually only entered by others in the course of love-making or comforting. Close proximity by non-intimates is generally experienced as uncomfortable or disconcerting (as in a crowded lift or train). Next is the *personal zone*, extending to approximately three feet from the body and within which most conversation takes place. The *social zone*—3 to 10 feet from the body—is the space where much of everyday life can 'properly' occur. Finally there is the *public zone*, which is beyond this. Hall calls these socially drawn, spatial distinctions 'proxemics'.

According to Hall, proxemic patterns vary cross-culturally. He believes it is possible by studying these patterns to demonstrate the otherwise hidden cultural framework which determines the structure of a people's perceptual world. Different cultures not only speak different languages but inhabit different sensory worlds. Moreover, men and women within any culture have different worlds; they learn to use their bodies in different ways because they are, by virtue of their gender roles, concerned with different things.

Hall's proxemics are useful in reminding us of attitudes towards personal space in both our society and others; attitudes which must inevitably form part of an individual's sexuality. In nursing we are frequently intruding into the personal space of patients. This may in itself be stressful, although people of different cultures will react differently. Research shows, for example, how many American patients may become angry to the point of violence when nurses do not ask permission before touching them in the course of taking observations of temperature, pulse and respiration. Those of Middle Eastern culture may react differently because of their different attitudes towards personal space—with the sex of the intruder being a more significant variable. Close physical proximity to patients may also be stressful for nurses.

Jourard (1971), for example, suggests the over-cheerful, detached bedside manner often found among nurses is, in part, a reaction to the physically intimate nature of the nurse/patient relationship. He sees it as representing a strategy for the prevention of emotionally or physically threatening behaviour from the patient.

Body-boundary and body products

As the discussion of space suggests, the location of one's body-boundary in relation to the rest of the world is somewhat arbitrary. What is taken to represent the body-boundary varies from one culture to another and is not always indicated by the skin. Generally the orifices of the body, such as the mouth or anus, are seen as gaps in body-boundary, with those body products that issue from them (such as breath, ear wax, menstrual blood, urine, faeces or semen) having special status due to their ambiguous nature; they are seen as neither part nor not-part of the body. Similar marginal status may also be given to other body products not associated with orifices, such as hair or nail clippings.

The status of body products varies cross-culturally. For example, those associated with the upper part of the body are seen by some as pure or even sacred (especially the breath) while those of the lower body are frequently perceived as impure or polluting. While these associations are clearer in some societies than others, (the Hindu caste system for example is in part based on the notions of purity and pollution), it cannot be assumed that body products have no such associations for those in Western society.

The association between body products and sexuality is little discussed but is nonetheless clear at erotic and non-erotic levels. Body odour, for instance, can be found sexually exciting. (Napoleon is said to have sent a message to Josephine from the battlefront saying 'Don't wash: coming home'.) Some people find urinating in a sexual context ('watersports') highly erotic. In common with other forms of eroticism it can also be used as a means of demonstrating power through humiliation. Processes such as defaecation may be pleasurable body experiences, if not frankly sexual, but as with other aspects of sexuality they can also be strongly associated with shame and therefore require strict privacy. Clearly the fact that nurses' work brings them in close contact with the body products of patients has some importance for the nurse-patient dynamic, especially where the patient is ashamed by loss of privacy. Yet surprisingly little work has been done concerning body products and, for example, their significance in the nurse-patient relationship.

This is also the case in connection with body-boundary, although it is obviously an important concept in our society. Helman (1978), for example, has shown this in very general terms. Working as a general practitioner in the suburbs of London, he finds that among the inhabitants of Stanmore, a sense of safety is associated with either the inside of the home or the inside of the body, while threats of danger come principally from without. Illnesses such as colds are thought to be the outcome of penetration of the body-boundary (chiefly the skin) by environmental forces such as damp, cold, or draughts, while 'bugs' or 'viruses' are seen as responsible for fever and gain access to the body through its various orifices. Defence is attempted by a strengthening of the body-boundary—often by the use of warm clothing, particularly to areas of skin thought more vulnerable to attack, such as the top of the head or back of the neck.

This is very different from understandings of body-boundary found in some other cultures. Among the Kwakiutl of North America for example, the skin may be strengthened by massage with oils or body painting. In some cultures (such as the Hopi of North America), threat is seen to come from within the body itself—more specifically from the individual's own emotions and actions (Postal 1965). Significantly, the role of emotion in the causation of illness such as ischaemic heart disease or cancer is now being considered in Western (primarily holistic) medicine.

According to Brown (1977), the concept of body-boundary is important in nursing as its procedures often involve a breach of such boundaries—for example, in giving injections or enemas, passing naso-gastric tubes, and taking cervical smears. All too often the symbolic meaning these actions may hold for the patient are given scant attention. The nurse, too, may feel her sense of body-boundary compromised by the close physical contact she has with her patients. The consideration of body-boundary becomes even more important if we recognise that the body-boundary (even in Western culture) does not strictly correspond with the limits of the body wall. It may, for example, include clothes and accessories that are habitually worn and this clearly has implications for patients whose familiar apparel is removed on admission to hospital.

In addition to cultural variation in the experience of bodily space, the everyday experience of the body and its boundary may vary with the effects of ill health. An individual who has undergone amputation of one leg may experience his body-boundary as continuing to include the area previously occupied by the leg. Some sufferers of schizophrenia or those under the influence of certain drugs appear to react to distant events as if they were directly affecting their bodies. Similarly distant events may be experienced as occurring within the body by those undergoing immense psychological trauma such as bereavement. As one interviewee told me:

'My mother was very ill. I knew she was dying and so did she. Hardly a minute would pass in which I didn't seem to think about her. . . . One morning I woke up and—it sounds crazy—but I felt I was somebody else. Even my sense of my body was different. I felt thin. Then it dawned on me—I was my mother! For a moment it was as if I was her.'

Most people can potentially experience what Fisher and Cleveland have called 'extreme versions of body-boundary contradictions' (1958). But as I suggested earlier, instead of there being one fixed reality, space—or our understanding of it—can be influenced by a number of factors, including social and psychological influences. It therefore comes as little surprise that in certain circumstances our sense of body-boundary is challenged to the extent that we may experience our own bodies as if they were others', or experience the body of another as if it were our own.

Body image

Closely linked to body-boundary is body image, the mental picture each person has of his or her own body. This internal image is formed by the interaction of bodily experiences, the effects of age and environmental influences (Brown 1977). According to Brown three principal levels of bodily experience contribute to body image. There is first of all our innermost bodily experience, originating from predominantly physiological processes. A person has a sense of the position of various parts of the body even if blind or, in a sighted person, if the eyes are closed. If your arm is moved while you watch, it is difficult to distinguish the sensation of movement from the knowledge of movement gained by sight. But with your eyes closed there is no difficulty in judging the finest movements. This 'muscle sense' depends to a large extent on nerve impulses from muscles, joints and tendons. We are usually quite unconscious of this 'sixth sense' by which the body knows itself, and judges the position of its parts and the relation of its parts to each other. This sense of the body has been called 'kinaesthesia' or more recently, 'proprioception'—the sense of the body as its own property. Other largely somatic influences on body image include hormonal changes (as in premenstrual syndrome) and changes in metabolism brought about by disease or drugs including alcohol. In addition, endocrine changes associated with fear and other emotions may alter body image, suggesting even the 'somatic' experience of the body is difficult to isolate as purely physiological.

Second, there are behavioural experiences influenced by age, bodily health, perception, personality and cognitive development. The child who has not yet thought to think abstractly, for instance, will experience her body differently from most adults. Similarly, an infant whose powers of visual fixation are relatively undeveloped has a narrower range of stimuli available to influence the formation of body image. Character traits such as aggression or passivity also influence the individual's experience of the body.

Third, topological experience—that is, experiences arising from superficial characteristics of the body—also contribute to body image. These include more physiological responses, such as the sensation of pressure. However they also encompass experiences that depend on social context—for example, whether a certain skin colour, particular sex, or body shape is valued above another.

The first theories of how body image is formed came from neurosurgeons in the 1930s, once they became aware that certain lesions of the cerebral cortex could affect the way individuals experienced their body. It was found, for example, that particular forms of brain damage might lead patients to deny the existence of particular parts of their body or to be unable to distinguish right from left. Other lesions might prevent the patient from 'knowing' he had some degree of paralysis. More dramatically, some caused patients to believe they possessed new body parts or even that the whole of their body had disappeared. These early theories attributed physiological causes only to body image. Later on, individual personality came to be acknowledged as an important element of body image. It was only comparatively recently, however, that external forces such as social values were also recognised as highly influential (Fisher and Cleveland *ibid*).

Certain changes in body form such as scarring, the effects of skin disease or stoma formation can affect the way a person experiences and 'visualises' his body. The body may be valued less because of disfigurement (what is known as negative body image). This is not surprising given social reactions to disfigurement. One research project sent non-disfigured individuals as their 'normal' selves to collect donations for charity by knocking on people's doors. The same volunteers also requested donations after being made-up to appear disfigured. Fewer people offered money to this second group, and those who did gave less. Other research shows that shop assistants assume disfigured customers are more likely to be dishonest than others, while in the United States, facial appearance has been found to influence the severity of punishment meted out to those convicted of crime (see Dixon 1985).

It is not only outward or visible changes that may affect body image. For example, the very presence of a malignant tumour may affect the way a person understands his or her body—perhaps seeing the body as a whole to be out of control or the site of conflict. The incontinent patient experiences a powerlessness related not simply to sphincter control but to a sense of the whole body being unorchestrated. Scars are well recognised as affecting the individual's concept of body image, but what is less clear is the way in which the idea of the removal of an organ and the intimate probing of a surgeon into what might be seen as one's innermost being may affect the individual's sense of both the body *and* self.

Just as the boundaries of the body may extend further than the skin, so body image extends beyond the physical body to include the clothes we wear and the smells we exude. The smells associated with an infected discharge, a fungating tumour or even with sexual intercourse may affect self-image and the value a person puts on his or her body. All too often, the devaluation associated with changed body image is significant enough to challenge the way in which the patient values herself as a person. Here, changed body image interacts with individual concepts of selfhood, potentially disrupting social relationships, including sexual ones.

Selfhood or self-concept

Selfhood, or self-concept, is central to sexuality. As Webb has pointed out, gender roles and gender identity both contribute to it (1985a). Working as a man in a female-dominated occupation, or *vice versa*, can affect self-concept. Doubt about some aspect of one-self as a sexual being may undermine self-concept. A sense of self is inseparable from a sense of the body, and the concept of selfhood extends beyond the body to include body-image and body-boundary, as well as non-bodily aspects of the individual which might be described as 'consciousness', 'being', 'spirit' or 'soul'.

The experience of infertility offers some insight into ways in which sexuality in its broadest sense can be intertwined with self-concept. According to Raphael-Leff (1986) few aspects of the personality remain unscathed by the deep sense of confusion, injustice and failure aroused by the knowledge of infertility. The infertile person has to question the birthright that most other people take for granted. This can lead to a loss of faith not only in the body's internal processes but also in the individual's very existence. Pfeffer and Woollett (1983) have documented some of the feelings that come with the realisation of infertility; how, for example, self-worth is chipped away by doubts about being a 'proper' man or woman.

The autobiographical account of Oliver Sacks, a neurologist who suffered severe injury in a climbing accident, demonstrates the intertwined nature of selfhood, body boundary and body image (1984). Sacks tore the muscles of his leg while running away from an enraged bull he encountered on his way up a mountain. Before the accident, Sacks saw himself as a highly active man. He 'worked out' regularly in a gymnasium. He enjoyed making physical demands on his body and experiencing its unfailing response. He felt himself to be at one with his body. This sense of his body changed rapidly with injury. After surgery to repair torn quadriceps he looks at his leg for the first time:

> 'In that instant, that very first encounter, *I knew not my leg*. It was utterly strange, not-mine, unfamiliar... I could no longer feel it as "mine", as part of me. ... It was absolutely *not-me*—and yet, impossibly, it was attached to me—and even more impossibly, "continuous" with me. ... The flesh beneath my fingers no longer seemed like flesh. ... The more I gazed at it

and handled it, the less it was "there", the more it became Nothing—and Nowhere.... It had no place in the world.' (*Ibid*: 47–9) (original emphasis)

Sacks experienced himself as an amputee, although objectively the leg was still there. He was, as he described it, an 'internal amputee'. He had lost his inner image of his leg—not only in the sense that he had lost all feeling *in* the leg but also much of his feeling *for* the leg. He could no longer remember how he had ever walked or run, although he had done both only a few days before, nor could he imagine how he could ever do these again or how he would ever *experience* his leg again. He found certainty of his body had come principally through action and now the uncertainty he experienced in the face of his non-functioning limb led to utter desolation—the 'essential aloneness of the patient'.

Sacks's dreams at this time were totally about his leg; his leg as unbending marble, as friable sand or—most terrifying of all—his leg as mist or just darkness, made of nothing at all. In order to come to terms with his new sense not only of part of his body but also of his being in the world, Sacks had to give up his identity as an active man and succumb to passivity. 'I found this humiliating at first, a mortification of my self, the active, *masculine* ordering self which I equated with my science, my self-respect, my mind' (*Ibid*: 79) (my emphasis). Recounting his dreams to other patients, he found his experience was in no sense unusual. Despite different injuries or pathologies, whether they were patients with strokes, with paraplegia or severe neuropathies, Sacks found all the patients he spoke to had similar dreams and were suffering from some body-image disorder. To varying extents they had all experienced alienation of parts of their body in which hands, feet etc. felt 'cut off', 'detached' or 'like nothing on earth'. None had been able to express these feelings to the medical staff. (Sacks does not refer to the involvement of the nursing staff.) Sacks points out that body image disturbance following peripheral injury or disease is common but not well discussed in the medical literature. He found on his return to work as a neurologist that all his patients who experienced a change in body image also underwent a profound questioning of their very being. This questioning was prompted by neuro-physiological events, but nevertheless involved fundamental change in their personal identity or selfhood.

Institutionalisation and loss of self-identity

An individual's sense of self can be seriously undermined not only by the effects of illness but also by those of institutionalisation accompanying illness. Brown (1966) points out that from the initial request after admission to get undressed and into bed, many patients are aware of a process which strips them of more than their clothing; their independence and self-identity are also peeled away. Patients are robbed of decision making and often treated as if they are children. Although with time some patients come to accept or even enjoy the withdrawal from all responsibility, others feel as if they have been forced into submission, their egos so deflated they cannot even protest.

Sanderson (1985), a health visitor, describes her brief experience of institutionalisation and its effects on her self-concept following meniscectomy. She became aware on admission of surrendering her independence, but also experienced a willingness to be carried along by the system. She found the regularity of the nursing routine reassuring. But long after the operation Sanderson remains disturbed that she cannot remember the first twenty-four post-operative hours—perhaps because in relinquishing awareness she also gave up control over her life. Two days after admission she found herself unable to make decisions and concerned that she would remain indecisive when she returned to work. She could just about make a choice from the hospital menu. In the space of a day she had moved from being active, independent and private to a dependency unknown to her since her childhood. Suddenly all her bodily functions were the object of scrutiny by strangers. Indeed one of her principle pre-operative concerns had been the dread of using bed pans. Unexpected menstruation was nearly the last straw. Despite good nursing care these ten days were so stressful that Sanderson felt totally drained when she left hospital—except that now she was without the protection of the institution she had come to depend on. Sanderson notes she found the whole experience taught her not only about the meaning of nursing but also something about herself.

If a few days in hospital can have such an effect on self-identity then clearly the effects of long-term institutionalisation may be profound. Goffman (1961) has shown something of these by demonstrating a regular sequence of changes experienced by many psychiatric patients in long-term care. He points out that although people admitted to psychiatric hospital vary widely in terms of the kind and degree of illness attributed to them, once they become in-patients they confront similar circumstances and tend to respond to these in similar ways, whatever their diagnosis. According to Goffman this uniformity of response provides some measure of the power of the institution.

One common reaction to institutionalisation is the adoption of a passive role, with a more or less blanket acceptance of treatment, house rules and routine. This stance is often viewed positively by staff, as such compliance makes their life so much easier. But passivity is not always in the patient's best interests, particularly if it adds to the loss of self-identity that is anyway experienced with ill health. In addition, sexual intimacy—one way in which identity and self-worth can be affirmed—is generally prohibited for those in long-term care (see also 'Institutionalisation', pp. 47–48 and 'Privacy', pp. 117–120).

Touch

Touch is closely linked with everything discussed in this section so far. Failure on the part of health workers to consider the significance of body-boundary through the indiscriminate use of touch, for example, can increase the alienation many patients experience as a result of institutionalisation. Alternatively, the appropriate use of touch can enhance body image and self-concept. Some patients respond to touch when all other attempts at communication are unsuccessful. Susannah Wright (1985) has described how, as a patient, touch seemed to awaken her will to recover.

Hall (*ibid*) bemoans the widespread lack of understanding of the deep significance of active touch. He sees touch as important in keeping the individual related to the world in which he or she lives. Barnett (1972a) notes that touch has been found to be one of the easiest and most elemental forms of communication for the human being, one which has never been entirely superseded by other processes such as speech. For Montagu (1978) touch is the mother of all the senses, being the earliest sensory system to become functional in all species. He finds the importance of the function of the skin has not gone unnoticed in common speech, with expressions such as 'rubbing someone up the wrong way', 'a soft touch', 'to get under one's skin', 'to be touchy', 'to be deeply touched' and so on indicating the everyday importance of touch.

Montagu is interested in the way tactile experience (or its absence) affects the development of behaviour. The effects of psychological stress on the skin (manifested for example by rashes, pimples etc.) are well recognised, but what interests Montagu is whether tactile sensations are necessary for physiological and psychological development and what may be the result of a lack of stimulation through the skin. Various studies he mentions have shown that in the animal world licking of the newborn is not only for cleanliness, but also essential for the stimulation of certain physiological functions. Without licking of the perineal area, for example, some young animals are susceptible to failure of the genito-urinary or gastro-intestinal systems. According to Montagu, although humans do not lick their newborns, a similar tactile stimulation of the human baby is achieved by the contractions of the uterus during labour.

Touch can be influenced by gender in that women in the West seem more ready to use expressive touch than men. This would seem to be linked to our earlier point that socialisation in this culture denies men ways of expressing emotion and dependency other than through genitalised sexuality. Age may also affect the use of touch. Barnett (ibid) and Goodykoontz (1979) show that patients aged 26 to 33 years are more frequently touched by nurses while patients over sixty-six years and pre-adolescents are touched least. (This is in contrast to what most nurses told me however; the majority of those I spoke to found it easier to touch older patients.) From research, it appears that older nurses tend to use touch less but this may simply be because the jobs most frequently occupied by older nurses involve less contact with patients anyway. According to Barnett the use of touch also varies within different specialties. She found touch was used most in paediatrics, intensive care and on the labour ward. It was least used in psychiatric nursing and on post-surgical and post-natal wards.

The patient's need to touch and be touched—whether by nurses, lovers, friends or relatives—is often increased because of the changes and fears they are experiencing. It is unfortunate that at the same time, the possibility of using touch is reduced because of the lack of privacy generally experienced in hospitals. (This problem will be elaborated in Chapter 7.)

The body politic and the nurse

While Chapter 1 showed something of the many facets of sexuality, this chapter has concentrated on personal understandings or experience of the body and/or self and how these are challenged by ill health and institutionalisation. As with other aspects of sexuality, much of this experience is socially influenced. This point is important because change—such as alteration of body image—can become slightly easier to deal with once it is recognised that ideal body form and emphasis on a perfect body are strongly shaped by the interests and influence of certain powerful sections of society, such as the advertising industry. Putting these values in context may help the patient not necessarily to accept change more wholeheartedly but to understand the problems he or she is experiencing in adapting to change. Nurses therefore need a good grasp of the ability of wider social forces to shape attitudes towards the body and self if they are to play a useful part in helping their patients to come to terms with change.

4

Ill health and sexual expression

Many aspects of sexuality should be borne in mind throughout patient care. Here and in the previous chapter, a distinction is drawn between erotic and non-erotic aspects simply as a means of organising the material. The distinction is really an artificial one, and is not at all clear-cut. As we saw earlier, erotic sex is more than a sexual act; it cannot be reduced to a number of physiological responses but is largely influenced by social factors and by the individual's general experience beyond any particular relationship or encounter. Some of the issues raised earlier must inevitably appear again here. Self-concept and body-image, for example, are closely interwoven with the phenomena of eroticism and desire; the effects of disease or surgery on these or other 'non-erotic' aspects of sexuality may lead in turn to a sexual problem such as loss of libido. Conversely, an explicitly sexual problem such as impotence may negatively affect non-erotic elements of sexuality such as self-concept or gender identity. The erotic and non-erotic therefore cannot be neatly disentangled.

Part of this chapter will look at the way in which ill health (using the term for convenience to include medical and surgical treatment of disease) may affect not only the physiology of sexual response, causing sexual problems, but also other apparently non-erotic aspects of sexuality, which in some way support the erotic. However, as stated earlier, this chapter deals only superficially with the specific effects of ill health on sexuality as this has been dealt with in detail elsewhere (see Further reading). Instead this chapter is more concerned with the way in which we actually think about sexual problems and whether, for example, current understandings of sexual function and dysfunction are adequate. It also considers the needs of those patients whose mode of sexual expression has been permanently affected by ill health and who may therefore wish drastically to alter their sexual behaviour or their role within a sexual relationship. This is not in itself an easy thing to do. But nurses should remember that many of the problems patients experience in this situation stem not only from the difficulties involved with change but also from lack of information and support. Moreover, problems are often compounded by the false assumptions that nurses and other health workers make about their patients' sexuality, by the limitations associated with well-defined gender roles and the restrictions imposed by institutionalisation.

Effects of ill health on sexuality

Just about any episode of ill health, from toothache to terminal illness, can affect some aspect of sexuality and the discussion below will cover just a few examples of how ill health in the form of disease, surgery, medication and radiotherapy or resulting in institutionalisation may affect both erotic and non-erotic sexuality. Perhaps more useful than any list or examples, however, is for each nurse to try to put herself in the position of her patient and try to imagine how she would feel about herself and her sexuality if she were suffering from the same complaint (such as a suppurating wound, menorrhagia or muscular sclerosis) or undergoing the same test (for example barium enema or subfertility investigations) that her patient has to tolerate.

Disease

One classic example of the effect of disease on sexuality is the experience of many male post-coronary patients for whom impotence is a common, albeit mostly temporary, condition. One of the principal sources of the problem lies in the fear of a further coronary or even sudden death brought on by sexual activity. Indeed, sex culminating in orgasm may well produce transient tachycardia or hyperventilation and while these resolve fairly rapidly after orgasm, they are still frightening reminders of the damage the heart has sustained. In addition it should not be forgotten that the heart is frequently thought of as the source of life and seat of emotions; it has symbolic as well as physiological significance for the individual. Damage to the heart therefore has fundamental implications for the individual's self-concept. Moreover, in Chapter 1 it was noted how sexual identity and gender identity are closely related. This can mean that for the male, post-coronary patient, impotence—in addition to other problems—will threaten his masculine identity and at the same time sabotage perhaps his only existing means of expressing or receiving tenderness or affection. (For a personal account which provides much insight into the way coronary heart disease may be experienced see Lear 1981.)

Surgery

The impact of surgery may be either fairly minimal (for example a neat scar after straightforward appendicectomy) or extremely difficult to come to terms with—as in the case of mastectomy. The effects of surgery on sexual functions *per se* can be wide-ranging. In some instances there may be actual physical damage which interferes with sexual response. Alternatively, surgical treatment may often have little direct effect on the physiology of sexual response but presents certain problems because of gender identity, or because the patient's overall self-image as a sexual being is affected. An obvious example of this is vasectomy, where loss of fertility may be confused with loss of potency or masculinity. Similarly, bladder or bowel surgery resulting in stoma formation may have an effect on continence and this can affect sexual expression by undermining confidence in the control of bodily functions as well as affecting body image. Both these effects may in turn cause patients to question their desirability.

Studies of patients with a permanent stoma have shown the intertwining of the physical and the psychological. For example, there appears to be a high incidence of impotence and ejaculatory problems among men with a stoma although whether this is the result of nerve damage during surgery or of psychological damage is difficult to assess (Eardley and Thornton 1976). If surgery is prompted by malignancy there may be additional problems postoperatively, with depression and anxiety that the disease is still present. Sex may be avoided because of fear of aggravating the disease or the feeling that it could be passed on to a partner. In any circumstance, surgery is often followed by a period of fatigue and anxiety, possibly resulting from the feeling that the body has been assaulted (especially if the site of surgery is an otherwise 'private' part of the body) or through the loss of identity and status associated with being a patient. These feelings, not surprisingly, may also affect sexual activity.

Medication

Sexual difficulties can also be induced by medication. Some drugs directly affect parts of the autonomic nervous system specifically associated with sexual response, causing problems with erection, vaginal lubrication, ejaculation or orgasm. Other drugs, such as corticosteroids, do not affect sexual physiology as such but may increase the patient's susceptibility to infection, causing either general malaise or secondary sexual problems (vaginal infections, for example). The sedative effects of some drugs (such as antihistamines) may reduce sexual desire. Sex hormones used therapeutically can affect fertility and secondary sexual characteristics (such as the development of gynaecomastia or change in hair distribution) and potentially undermine gender identity and self-concept.

Cytotoxic drugs may cause amenorrhoea or reduced spermatogenesis. Patients taking these drugs may have no immediate interest in reproduction but nonetheless may feel it important to be able to view themselves as potentially fertile. The absence of menstruation may be an additional sign for women not only that their fertility or perhaps their femininity is in some way threatened but also that their whole body is not functioning normally. The effect of hair loss or weight loss as a result of some forms of chemotherapy may also have far-reaching effects on self-image for both men and women. Nausea and vomiting as a result of gastrointestinal toxicity will invariably affect sexual interest while some chemotherapy—or drugs such as narcotics used in conjunction with cytotoxics—may reduce libido more directly. Finally, because of drug-induced immunosuppression, patients receiving chemotherapy may be nursed in isolation or made subject to various forms of protection from visitors and health workers. Not only does this place an embargo on sexual activity with others, but non-erotic needs, such as the need to touch and be touched, are also unfulfilled. Furthermore, after treatment is discontinued there may be difficulties in adjusting to non-isolation.

Radiotherapy

Some radiotherapy regimes are more detrimental to aspects of sexual activity than the alternative treatments of surgery or chemotherapy. Gastrointestinal mucosa are especially sensitive to radiation and depending on the area being treated, oral-genital or oral-anal sex may be limited by ulceration. Depending on the degree of bone marrow irradiation, there may be a significant decrease in white blood cells and platelets, predisposing the patient to infection or haemorrhage following penetrative or oral sex. Body image changes can occur as a result of change in appearance of the skin where radiotherapy causes erythema, desquamation or, rarely, radiation burns. Fear of damage to the skin together with advice to avoid any irritation or friction to the skin's surface may lead to an avoidance of sexual activity. Additionally, radiotherapy may cause nausea, tiredness or general malaise—all contributing to a reduced interest in communication including sexual expressiveness.

Institutionalisation

Institutionalisation can either be long- or short-term. Much of what is covered in this book will be relevant to those in long-term care. In addition special aspects such as the sexual needs of the severely disabled or the rights of mentally handicapped people to sexual relationships raise very specific issues. For example, to what extent should nurses actively assist their disabled patients in finding sexual satisfaction? What is the role of the nurse *vis-à-vis* the right of handicapped patients to sexual expressiveness? These areas remain highly controversial and unfortunately cannot be dealt with adequately here. Nurses working with people in long-term care may find the 'Further reading' suggested at the end of the chapter useful. They can also contact SPOD, MIND and MENCAP for further information.

In the case of relatively short-term institutionalisation, we have already seen how simply becoming a patient can affect sexuality (see p. 39). In addition to this the individual may be affected by loss of income once sickness benefits expire, or suffer reduced social status if unemployment results from ill health, and such changes can result in an undermining of self-image. Hospitalisation may also mean additional responsibilities and domestic chores for partners and possible restrictions on *their* activities. These effects are enough to place a strain on any relationship but as if this were not enough, the effects of illness and any accompanying change of role may also affect sexual self-image. Moreover, separation from a sexual partner or partners through hospitalisation restricts sexual expression and can result in frustration and resentment. The continuity of a relationship may be disrupted, and this in itself can lead to sexual difficulties. At the same time, the implications of illness may also prompt fears for the future sex role of the individual.

Sexual function and dysfunction

So far, discussion of the patient's sexuality has been couched in terms of erotic and non-erotic forms of sexuality and their interrelatedness. I have not talked of 'sexual dysfunction' as a result of ill health. This is because there are certain problems and assumptions within current definitions of sexual function and dysfunction which I believe should prevent these terms from being automatically applied in all contexts.

The term 'sexual function' generally refers to sexual behaviour or events corresponding to the four stages of 'sexual response' defined by Masters and Johnson (see pp. 11–12). Conversely, 'sexual dysfunction' refers, by and large, to the disruption of the pattern of this response as a result of physiological or psychological problems. Deviation from this model of response is generally assumed to be unhealthy or sexually unfulfilling.

Since the concept of sexual dysfunction is based on a narrow understanding of normal sexual function, the forms sexual dysfunction may take are also fairly limited. Male sexual dysfunction is indicated by problems with erection, libido, premature ejaculation or absence of orgasm or ejaculation. Female sexual dysfunction is characterised either by total absence or secondary loss of libido, anorgasmia (absence of orgasm) or vaginismus (spasm of vaginal muscles preventing penetration). In addition to these problems there may be 'joint dysfunction'—in other words, difficulties may be experienced by both partners in a relationship, with the other person's problems tending to reinforce the difficulty each experiences.

However, while the forms of sexual function are fairly limited, the causes are many. They include increased age, generalised illness, specific disease (for example, diabetes), genital abnormalities, psychiatric disorders such as depression, or the effects of certain drugs. Non-physical causes include personal problems such as poor self-esteem, or interpersonal difficulties (for instance conflict within a relationship). Finally, lack of knowledge about the body and 'situational' causes such as lack of privacy or fear of pregnancy may also be involved. In other words, psychological or organic problems become expressed as specific forms of sexual difficulty. Significantly *anyone* can have a sexual problem; it is not necessary to be physically ill or institutionalised for some form of sexual dysfunction to develop.

It is not possible here to go into all the treatments of sexual dysfunction in any depth but it is necessary to enlarge a little on psychosexual therapy. The main reason for this is that the general nurse should have some idea of the methods and scope of psychosexual therapy in order to recognise when it is appropriate to refer a patient with a sexual problem and what therapy might involve.

Psychosexual therapy includes a number of approaches such as the teaching of sexual technique (for instance, the importance of foreplay for some women), or modified psychotherapy in which, for example, the power dynamic of a relationship may be explored and its effects on the couple's sexual behaviour understood. By and large it is couples rather than individuals who are treated. In therapy based on Masters' and Johnson's work, sexual response is seen as a natural function which can be upset by problems such as physical stress or anxiety. Dysfunctions such as vaginismus or premature ejaculation are viewed as conditioned reflex responses to such problems which can be reconditioned. For this, couples may be trained in practical intervention—such as the use of vaginal dilators in the case of vaginismus or the 'squeeze technique' to temporarily inhibit orgasm in persistent premature ejaculation (for more details see 'Further reading').

There are several schools of thought within psychosexual therapy; ideally it should not be treated as a single body of ideas. However, in order to indicate where this form of therapy may be appropriate it is necessary to look at its limitations and, in doing so, for the sake of brevity, I tend to treat the many approaches within psychosexual work as a homogeneous system. In the following argument I do not mean to be unduly hard on the psychosexual therapist. It must be remembered that many people have benefited enormously from this form of treatment. I merely wish to indicate its limitations so that nurses may have a clearer picture of where specialist intervention of this sort may be helpful. It is also useful here to start considering the way in which the skills of the general nurse can, in some instances, be more appropriate than those of the specialist or, in other situations, complement the work of the psychosexual counsellor. (This point will be developed more in Chapter 9.)

The limitations of psychosexual therapy

Some of the limitations of psychosexual therapy result from the poor understanding of sexuality which underlies its practice. In common with many other theories, psychosexual theory all too often assumes 'sex' to be heterosexual, penile-vaginal intercourse leading to orgasm—even though this form of sexual activity may be undesirable, unavailable or impossible for many people. Homosexuality, for example, is often treated if not exactly as a form of sexual dysfunction then certainly as a sexual problem (see for example Hesford and Bhanji on homosexuality as 'deviation' (1986)). Some authorities in this field even see the distinction between sexuality in general and sexual dysfunction as increasingly blurred. For example, some training courses claiming to deal with human sexuality are predominantly concerned with enabling course participants to act as psychosexual counsellors and to treat sexual dysfunction. The point has to be made that sexuality is not, in itself, a problem!

The emphasis of psychosexual treatment is, by and large, towards the creation or restoration of sexual function—but what is at issue is a very specific idea of sexual function, that is, one consistent with Masters' and Johnson's model of sexual response. One of the problems with this is that the model becomes mistaken for reality. As I said in Chapter 1, Masters and Johnson only intended the four stages of sexual response they described to be seen as a simplification of human experience, not as a blueprint. What is generally assumed, though, is that people engaging in sex should pass in proper sequence from one state of arousal to another and finish off with one or more orgasms.

One consequence of this idea is that sexual expression becomes a type of performance and that this can be objectively rated as successful or otherwise. Sex becomes value-laden. 'Good sex', like a good play, is well structured with orgasm as the grand finale and the resolution phase as curtain call. Implicit judgement is indicated by the very language used by some writers in the psychosexual field and can be found, for example, in Hesford's and Bhanji's definition of sexual dysfunction as 'a *deficit* of sexual performance' or Glover's description of anorgasmia as 'the *failure to acheive* orgasm' (1985) (my emphasis).

The problem with this process is that objective assessments of sexual function tend to be given priority over the *meaning* sex has for the individual—even though this personal meaning will often influence the way in which sexual pleasure is actually experienced. Such experience moreover may not conform to the Masters and Johnson model of sexual response. All too often, 'sexual function' is understood as a single-stranded and essentially biologically-determined pattern of sexual response; there is no way of incorporating behavioural variation (such as excitement without orgasm) other than as sexual dysfunction. This ultimately means that forms of psychosexual therapy strongly dependent on this model of sexual response have a limited usefulness for those who do not or cannot conform to this 'painting by numbers' approach to sexual expression.

It also suggests that, just as 'sexual function' needs to be rethought and variation in sexual response acknowledged, so what is meant by 'sexual dysfunction' should be reconsidered. Any useful definition of 'sexual dysfunction' should not be restricted to problems in the four stages of sexual response defined by Masters and Johnson but should refer to any problem *defined by the patient* as a sexual problem.

Some sexual problems, for example, those arising directly from ill health, fall outside the standard definition of sexual dysfunction and consequently outside the framework of many forms of psychosexual therapy. I am thinking particularly of those instances where ill health has led to permanent restrictions on previous forms of sexual expression. In these cases there is very often a lack of support and information for patients. This could be provided by the general nurse if she has been adequately trained. (For a discussion of the role of the nurse in basic sexual health care, sexual adjustment and psychosexual therapy see Chapter 9.)

Restrictions on sexual expression

Sexual activity can be modified in a number of ways by ill health. In some instances, the entire mode of sexual expression usually available to the patient is undermined. For some people with long-term disabilities, sexual activity can be affected because it requires advance planning. Urinary catheters, for example, may need to be removed or, with supra-pubic catheters, securely taped in place. Those using intermittent catheterisation to maintain continence may need to empty the bladder before sex. Stoma bags may need to be changed to avoid leakage. Some preparations involve considerable foresight. For instance for those in chronic pain, analgesia may need to be taken in advance. Where spasticity occurs (as with some forms of spinal cord injury) this may not only determine the type of sexual practice or position adopted but may also require medication before sexual activity is possible. The post-coronary patient may be advised in some instances to take beta-blockers one hour before sex where palpitations have occurred, or to use a prophylactic coronary dilator five to ten minutes before sexual activity, to prevent angina (Thompson and Cordle 1986).

In some cases, ill health and its results may influence the actual form of sexual expression. For the person who has suffered a stroke, cutaneous hypersensitivity or loss of sensation can affect sexual arousal and the patient and any partner have to rediscover what kind of touching is pleasurable and what is unpleasant (Riley 1986). A high proportion of people suffering from arthritis experience some degree of sexual difficulty arising from the pain, reduced joint movement, deformity and disability associated with the disease (Hamilton 1976). For the woman, arthritis of the hip may prevent the conventional 'missionary' position of heterosexual intercourse. Indeed some surgeons have been known to undertake total hip replacement largely because of this aspect of arthritic disability. But as Hamilton points out, such measures are not always the best solution. Alternative positions for intercourse which take the strain off painful joints—with, for example, the affected partner standing, sitting or kneeling—should be considered, or less physically demanding alternatives to sexual intercourse could be sought, such as oral-genital sex or mutual masturbation.

There are some instances where the patient is compelled to find an entirely different mode of sexual expression if he or she is to continue sexual activity. For example, apart from drastically affecting body-image, radical vulvectomy results in extensive alteration of anatomy and physiology. In addition to the vulva, the vagina and bowel may be affected—especially where there are metastases—to the extent that vaginal or anal penetration may no longer be possible. Clitoral tissue may also be removed and this may influence orgasmic response. The effects of pelvic exenteration may be even more severe. Here most of the pelvic organs (including the vagina) are generally removed, necessitating the formation of an artificial bladder and/or colostomy. Adaptation in terms of sexual identity depends on a number of factors. Depression and emotional trauma are high among these patients. One study (Brown *et al.* 1972) followed fifteen women over a three-year period following this type of surgery and found a very varied picture. Seventy-three per cent of the women had no interest in sex at the time of the study (compared to 13 per cent pre-operatively). Thirty-eight per cent had tried 'unusual sexual practices' although what this meant or the role played by any partner was not discussed in the report. Some women masturbated by manipulating the scar tissue of the mons veneris and one woman digitally manipulated her ileostomy which had become eroticised. (The mucocutaneous junction is similar to that of the mouth, genitals and anus.)

Abdo-perineal resection or proctocolectomy can also have drastic effects on sexual expression and not only because of altered body image. Female patients may suffer dyspareunia (pain on intercourse) although this is usually only temporary. As previously mentioned, damage to nerve pathways can in some cases lead to permanent impotence for male patients, particularly where surgery was undertaken for malignancy. For homosexual men who participate in anal intercourse the loss of the anus and rectum also removes a major source of pleasure and possibly sexual identity. In some instances the stoma has been used as an alternative site for penetration but this can cause damage.

People with a confirmed diagnosis of AIDS or testing positive for antibodies to the AIDS virus are encouraged to make restrictions on sexual activity in order to protect their sexual contacts and to protect themselves against the risk of further infection. Such restrictions include a limitation on the number of sexual partners and the avoidance of anal or vaginal intercourse. Fellatio (oral-penile sex) or oral-anal contact are also considered risky and best avoided. Other sexual activities such as mutual masturbation and body rubbing are thought to be relatively safe but may involve quite a shift of sexual orientation. In addition, all those *at risk* of acquiring the AIDS virus (now a sizeable proportion of the general population) are being urged to consider their sexual practices. They too are being asked to reduce their number of sexual partners, to use a condom (this alone may represent something of a challenge to those unused to such manoeuvres) or to avoid penetrative sex. (For more details about safer sexual practices see leaflets from the Terrence Higgins Trust and Health Education Authority: Further reading.)

To give a final example, radical treatment for cancer involving the male genitalia—such as penectomy (removal of the penis) has obvious implications for many forms of sexual expression. Men who have undergone penectomy are often deeply ashamed of their changed body appearance and experience a loss of both masculinity and social identity. In addition to this, where sexual expression has focused on penetration, a major source of sexual pleasure has been lost. Considering the social and sexual importance of the penis it is not surprising that there is a relatively high incidence of suicide following this type of surgery.

In these more extreme forms of limitation on sexual expression, and in those instances where erotic sexuality is less drastically modified by the effects of ill health, the patient's identity as a sexual being can be maintained by the introduction of new sexual practices or a different sexual emphasis (for example, one less centred on orgasm or penetration).

For such changes to occur, a great deal will depend on the nature of any sexual relationship existing before ill health and on the present attitude of the patient and (where present) partner. It is extremely difficult for many people deliberately to change the way they relate sexually—either to others or to themselves. Within a sexual relationship such changes can have far-reaching implications by challenging gender roles or altering the balance of forces or power structure that exists within the relationship. For some—perhaps because of these implications or because of objections on religious grounds—alternative practices will prove unacceptable. For others, the process of rediscovering sexual needs and pleasures may mean not only the continuation but the deepening of their sexual relationships. A great deal also depends on the kind of information and support the patient receives. Nurses can play an important role here but much will depend on their attitude and ability to free themselves from assumptions about their patients' sexuality.

Limiting assumptions

I want to highlight three common assumptions which may be found as frequently among nurses as other members of the population. These concern sexual preference, sexual practice and whether the patient is considered to be a sexual being in the first place.

The assumption of heterosexuality

Erotic sexuality is generally assumed to be essentially concerned with heterosexuality. This view rests on two premises. The first is that heterosexuality is in some way more 'natural' than other forms of sexuality. Secondly, sexual preference and sexual desire are assumed to be fixed at a certain point, such as birth or puberty, and are subsequently unchanging. Both beliefs have been countered by the work of Kinsey and other sexologists who suggest that sexuality represents a continuum. At one end of the scale is exclusive heterosexuality and at the other, exlcusive homosexuality—with most people's proclivities falling somewhere between these two points (that is, either more or less homosexual, more or less bisexual or more or less heterosexual).

While heterosexuality is undoubtedly the social norm in Western culture, its social acceptability says very little about most people's actual sexual desire, only about expected behaviour. Cross-culturally, the incidence of homosexuality and bisexuality varies quite independently of official attitudes. It may be an unusual practice where it is prohibited and usual where it is endorsed. On the other hand though, it can be common in some cultures where it is forbidden or even uncommon where it is sanctioned (Whitehead 1981). This indicates that sexual preference is not the automatic outcome of human biology, psychology or culture, but as stated in Chapter 1, is also influenced by personal choice.

One of the dangers of assuming heterosexual orientation is that specific, health-related needs of non-heterosexual patients will be neglected by nurses. The informational needs of a male homo-sexual undergoing abdo-perineal resection, for example, may be very different from those of a heterosexual male having the same operation. One gay man has described how the peri-anal abscesses associated with inflammatory bowel disease considerably limited his sexual activity as well as damaging his whole sexual and social self-image (Cant 1985). But his suffering was made worse because of the difficulty of obtaining information specifically relevant to his mode of sexual expression. Eventually his disease became so debilitating that he was advised to have his rectum and colon removed. It seemed that freedom from chronic and excruciating pain was to be at the price of his sexual identity; he felt that, with the removal of his rectum, he would become a 'sexual dinosaur'. Fortunately, at this point this patient found help through the Ileostomy Association who put him in touch with other gay men who *had* agreed to this type of surgery and who could reassure him of its advantages. He went ahead with the operation and, at the time of writing, felt better than he had for years, partly because he was well enough to experience himself as a sexual being again.

Although Cant does not say so explicitly, it would seem his search for information and support was a solitary one—he does not mention, for example, help from medical or nursing staff and although his story has a happy ending, not everyone would be so self-motivated and persistent. Cant indicates that he had 'come out' as a homosexual and was therefore able actively to search for help and information. The situation must be even more difficult for those homosexuals who feel unable to be open about their sexual preferences.

The intercourse assumption

Alongside the 'heterosexuality assumption' exists the 'intercourse assumption'. This takes for granted that 'sex' equals penile-vaginal penetration, so ignoring other forms of sexual expression such as masturbation, oral-genital sex, manual penetration, extragenital stimulation or fantasy. Where male homosexuality *is* acknowledged it is perceived just as narrowly as focusing on penile-anal penetration. Lesbianism seems to have escaped such rigid definition but, I suspect, only because non-lesbians by and large cannot imagine what is possible without men!

One of the drawbacks of the intercourse assumption is that

what is understood by the term 'sex' can have important implications for the successful treatment of a number of diseases. For
example, in the case of cystitis (most commonly found among
women) the health worker often recommends that there should be
'no sex' until treatment is completed. Just what is prohibited may
be unclear to patient and health worker alike. Generally, restrictions are suggested because vaginal penetration may cause increased irritation of the vagina and urethra with the possibility of
introducing more harmful bacteria. But this explanation provides
no reason for why other forms of sexual expression should be
avoided. Conversely, one of the main causes of vaginitis—*Candida
albicans*—can also infect the tongue and buccal mucosa. Here then
a simple prohibition of 'sex' (given that this is generally taken to
mean penile-vaginal intercourse) is insufficient to prevent infection of a partner as this may occur through oral-genital sex
(Whatley 1986).

Wilmer (1981), relating her experience as a patient, provides
another example of the intercourse assumption. Following hysterectomy she was given the cursory advice 'No sex until your next
appointment'. This she assumed (and she was probably right) to
mean sexual intercourse, i.e. penetrative sex. She therefore did not
think she would be contravening this advice when she masturbated five weeks after leaving hospital. Subsequently she began to
bleed and although the loss was slight it was unexpected and
therefore quite frightening. As Wilmer says, such distress could
have been avoided if she had been given more comprehensive
advice.

Finally there are some circumstances where no form of sexual
activity is assumed for the most negative of reasons. This is most
clearly the case in relation to age.

Assumptions about age

According to some writers (e.g. Krajicek 1982) sexuality begins
before birth, existing for the fetus *in utero*. Children are born with
sexual feelings which are developed by activities such as rocking,
stroking or fondling. Certainly the infant is sexually curious,
exploring its body at an early age and learning that touching the
genitals is pleasurable. Sexuality is also influenced by parental
attitudes for example towards toilet training or playing with the

genitals. It was not until relatively recently—perhaps not until the work of Freud—that there was any recognition of children's sexuality, and even now, this recognition is not widespread. Alternatively children's grasp of gender role—whether, for example, they enjoy playing with dolls or guns—may be mistakenly described as early sexuality. This confusion between gender and sexuality can have implications for the very young patient; their social development may be assessed yet their sexual development ignored. For children, a long stay in hospital can affect relationships with both parents and peers, and ultimately influence sexual development. In addition, opportunities for children to learn experimentally about their bodies are restricted by hospitalisation and, very often, by the attitudes of health workers. Masturbation, for example, despite being a fundamentally important way of beginning to understand one's sexuality, is generally discouraged even where the child has privacy.

At the other end of the age scale, the sexuality of the elderly is not widely recognised. Western society is primarily youth- and work-oriented. Just as this orientation has isolated many elderly people from adequate income and meaningful social activity, it has also led to a denial of the elderly as sexual beings (Yeaworth and Friedman 1975). This attitude is endorsed by many 'folk' beliefs about sex and age—for instance that loss of semen represents loss of strength and that sexual abstinence promotes long life. It is not just that people ignore the sexuality of the elderly—there is actually a negative attitude towards it. The concept of masturbation in childhood, for example, is vaguely tolerated. It is seen as natural—if a little *too* natural!—but the practice of masturbation by the elderly is generally regarded as sick.

Undoubtedly the ageing process does have some effect on sexual practice. The five senses, which can all play a role in sexual expression, generally become less acute with age. The literature which does consider the effects of ageing on sexual function again tends to assume heterosexual activity and emphasises penile-vaginal intercourse. It therefore concentrates on the physiological response associated with penetration. In post-menopausal women, for instance, it is noted there is a decrease in the potential of the vagina for expansion, and natural lubrication may be reduced. In the male, full erection takes more time. So too does ejaculation (not always a bad thing!). The resolution phase of sexual response described by Masters and Johnson may also be longer, with an inability to redevelop an erection for up to twenty-four hours for some men over fifty.

The point of much of this literature is to demonstrate that for the majority, the potential for sexual expression continues into old age. Much of it fails to make the point though that 'sex' is more than penile-vaginal penetration or that alternatives to penile-vaginal penetration may be increasingly practised with advancing years. Contrary to the stereotype created of the elderly, people are not necessarily increasingly inflexible as they get older—at least about modes of sexual expression. A significant proportion of men, for example, experience homosexual sex for the first time after the age of sixty (McCarey 1973). I am not aware of similar findings about women but it would seem surprising if there were no similar trend, especially remembering that more women than men survive into old age. Finally Masters and Johnson have found there is a 50 per cent chance of resolving sexual difficulties experienced by people over the age of fifty—even if the problems have existed for twenty-five years or more.

As Dolan (1985) points out, sexuality—ranging from the need for sexual intercourse to the need to be touched—is as central to the elderly as it is for any other group and to ignore this is to ignore an important element of nursing care. She describes how a well-oriented eighty-three year old female patient suddenly developed urinary incontinence. After ruling out other causes it was eventually elicited that the patient was deliberately incontinent in order to experience the touch and attention that came with being cleaned up afterwards. The problem of incontinence stopped when her needs were recognised and she was given more physical attention such as more frequent back rubs.

Discussion and information are also important aspects of nursing care of the elderly prior to treatment such as radiotherapy or surgery. Many gynaecologists, for example, without discussion and assuming their elderly patients to be celibate, tighten the vagina during a repair operation to the extent that penetrative sex is no longer possible. Or vaginal irradiation is prescribed without informing the patient that it may carry the risk of vaginal stenosis and reduced lubrication. The provision of information regarding these potential side effects, together with details of remedial measures (such as the early use of mechanical dilatation and topical oestrogen where penetrative sex is desired) can make all the difference between the end or the continuation of the patient's (and any partner's) normal sex life. All too often though, the elderly patient is not provided with such information; it is assumed to be irrelevant.

Previous chapters have given some indication of the range of issues which may be covered by the term 'the patient's sexuality' and the ways in which sexuality can be affected by ill health. They also began to look at the *potential* role of the nurse in helping patients to come to terms with effects of ill health on sexuality. The extent to which nurses are *actually* involved in this work—and indeed, whether it is fair to expect them to become involved at all—will be discussed over the following chapters.

Further reading

Bullard D. and Knight S. eds (1982). *Sexuality and Physical Disability: Personal Perspectives*. St Louis: Mosby.

Craft A. and Craft M. (1979). *Handicapped Married Couples*. London: Routledge & Kegan Paul.

Greengross W. (1976). *Entitled to Love: The Sexual and Emotional Needs of the Handicapped*. London: Malaby Press.

Kaplan H. (1976). *The Illustrated Manual of Sex Therapy*. London: Souvenir Press.

Kolodny R., Masters W., Johnson V. and Biggs M. (1979). *The Textbook of Human Sexuality for Nurses*. Boston: Little, Brown & Co.

Mooney T., Cole M. and Chilgren R. (1975). *Sexual Options for Paraplegics and Quadriplegics*. Boston: Little, Brown & Co.

Stanley K. (1985). In-patients' Human Rights. *Nursing Mirror* Jan. 16, Vol. 160 (**3**): 21–3.

Wadleigh P. (1982). Sexual dysfunction and therapeutic approaches. In *Human Sexuality in Nursing Process*. (Lion E., ed.). New York: John Wiley & Son.

AIDS

Health Education Authority leaflet: *AIDS: What everybody needs to know*. Published by AIDS Unit, Department of Health, 1986. Copies available from Dept A., P.O. Box 100, Milton Keynes, MK1 1TX.

Terrence Higgins Trust leaflets, *Safe Sex* and *AIDS and HTLV III: Medical Briefing*. Copies available from The Terrence Higgins Trust, BM AIDS, London WC1N 3XX.
AIDS Briefing. (1987). *New Scientist* **113**(1553):36–59.

Organisations

Ileostomy Association. Amblehurst House, Woking, Surrey GU24 8P2.
MENCAP. 123 Golden Lane, London EC1.
MIND. 22 Harley Street, London WIN 2ED.
SPOD (Sexual and Personal Relations of the Disabled). 286 Camden Road, London N7 0BJ.

5

Nursing and gender

Sexuality in its broadest sense (including, for example, gender-role expectations) has had an enormous impact on the development of nursing and on the delivery of nursing care. This chapter looks first at the effect of our 'sexual division of labour', and how definitions of women's and men's capabilities have historically helped to determine what is considered an appropriate role for the nurse, and goes on to examine the way in which nursing theory itself is strongly and negatively influenced by an approach built, in part, on unquestioned gender roles.

The sexual division of labour

In Chapter 1 we saw how in all societies to varying degrees, work is divided between the sexes on the basis of gender roles. Some tasks are allocated principally or exclusively to women, others to men, although this does not rule out the possibility that some work may be undertaken by both sexes (Mackintosh 1981). What is seen as 'appropriate' work for either sex, however, is far from standard cross-culturally, and far from unchanging in any one culture; as societies undergo change and the nature of work changes, so the distribution of work between men and women may also change. This helps to demonstrate that a sexual division of labour is linked to social rather than biological factors.

In Western society a sexual division of labour exists in both waged and non-waged work. In the domestic sphere, childcare, cooking, housework and other domestic tasks are primarily undertaken by women and are generally undervalued in comparison with the occasional domestic activities that may be performed by men, such as lawn-mowing or redecorating. At the same time, the extent of women's responsibilities in the domestic sphere very often restricts their involvement in other areas such as waged employment. The full-time housewife usually has no financial autonomy and little voice in the public sphere. She is in a poor position to influence or to challenge the social relations that underlie the sexual division of labour. In other words, the sexual division of labour not only expresses the subordinate position of women but also helps to perpetuate it.

Where both women and men work for wages, the sexual division of labour finds women segregated into occupations which are typically lower paid, coming lower in an overall hierarchy of authority and with relatively poor conditions of work—like nursing!

Women and nursing

It is no accident that women constitute the majority of the nursing workforce and that the majority of doctors have, until very recently, been men. In order to understand the present division of labour within health care, the polarisation between caring and curing and the respective identification of women and men with these different activities, it is necessary briefly to look at the historical development of nursing and medicine.

In the thirteenth century in Britain, the health needs of the majority of the population were served by lay healers of both sexes, who amalgamated the roles of present-day nurses and doctors; there was no split between caring and curing. According to Ehrenreich and English (1973) lay healers of this period were empiricists; they believed in trial and error, cause and effect. This was the very opposite of the Church's position, which opposed the value of the material world, distrusting any emphasis on knowledge obtained via the senses. The Church attacked the 'magic' of the lay healer through the institution of the witch hunt. Clearly other issues were involved. Approximately 85 per cent of 'witches' denounced and punished by the Church were women and in addition to being charged with the use of healing and midwifery skills, female witches were accused of committing sexual crimes against men and of possessing a 'female sexuality'. As Ehrenreich and English point out, the persecution of witches represented not only the anti-empiricist but also the anti-sexual obsessions of the Church at this time.

The era of witch hunting coincided with the emergence of a new all-male medical profession based on a university training which excluded women, and was strongly controlled by the Church. It was not possible to practise medicine without a priest in attendance and doctors could not treat patients who refused confession.

At the same time, legislation made the practice of lay healing illegal, although these laws were for the most part impossible to endorse. Because doctors served a different (and wealthier) clientele, the majority of lay healers represented little threat to the new medical establishment, so their prosecution was not important. However, *literate* women who had previously attended the affluent merchant class did initially represent a challenge to the new profession and it was these women who were actively prosecuted if they attempted to work as healers. In contrast, pregnancy and childbirth remained the province of female traditional midwives until at least the seventeenth century. Then male practitioners began not only to infiltrate this sphere but also to restrict the work of midwives by promoting the use of 'surgical instruments', such as forceps, which women were legally barred from using.

Despite these sexual politics, women have a long tradition of health care. However, nursing as organised, paid employment is a comparatively recent occupation, largely coinciding with the development of a hospital-based health care system. With this there was a shift from the care of the sick by their families at home to the removal of the 'patient' into hospital. Foucault (1973) suggests this move came about because the requirements of the new science of medicine coincided with those of the political ideology of the time; both desired a greater ease of observation or surveillance.

Jewson (1976) describes this process as a move from what he calls 'bedside medicine'—where the sick person was regarded as a whole entity whose history rather than whose body had to be carefully examined—to 'hospital medicine', which saw the sick person more as a collection of interrelated organs. With bedside medicine, doctors competed amongst themselves for the patronage of the patient, who was usually wealthy and to some extent able to control the method of medical investigation, whereas with hospital medicine, the sick person became relatively powerless in relation to the doctor. Not only was the patient generally of a lower social class than the doctor but the doctor's actions were principally controlled by the senior members of his profession, rather than by his client.

The role of nursing in this process has been given scant attention. As Versluysen (1980) points out, the history of health care is generally taken to be the same as the history of medicine. She argues that despite women's central role in health care through the ages, they are represented by historians as either 'old wives' (meaning well-intentioned but superstitious 'hags'), exceptional heroines, or ministering angels; in other words as surrounded by a mystical aura which sharply contrasted with the 'rationality' of medical men. As Versluysen says, these stereotypes provide little information about women's historical role in health care although they say plenty about social attitudes towards women among historians. Nightingale, for example, is characterised as 'The Lady with the Lamp', moving among her adoring patients in the Crimea, the very paragon of tenderness and compassion. Her intellectual and political interests—such as her work on medical statistics, Imperial India and the British Army Medical Corps, or her manipulation of the presiding Cabinet of the day, are largely ignored. These activities did not fit the stereotype of the upper-class Victorian woman, or the image of femininity at the time. Moreover, as Whittaker and Olesen (1978) argue, these activities remain largely unacceptable for women in our society. Therefore in hospital training schools where the principle of hierarchy still reigns and nurses are made subordinate to doctors, Nightingale's intellectual activities are suppressed. The same authors argue that in university nursing courses, the emphasis on the nurse as a co-member of the health care team (of which the doctor is but another member) and the importance placed on intellectual curiosity again influences the portrayal of the figure of Nightingale, but this time her academic achievements are emphasised while other aspects of her work are played down. What is clear is that Nightingale thought that to be a good nurse is to be a good woman (although she also said that the elements of nursing are all but unknown). In her day, women were seen to possess *biological* characteristics, such as an innate ability to nurture, which made them the ideal carers for the sick. At the same time, these characteristics also made them the best attendants for the doctor. According to Ehrenreich and English, modern nursing (that is, post-Nightingale) remains a product of the social circumstances of unmarried, upper-class Victorian women who sought refuge from a life of enforced leisure. The ideal nurse was a transformation of the ideal lady. Relieved of her reproductive responsibilities, she was transposed from domestic life to hospital life, taking with her a wifely obedience to the doctor (who was in turn the perfect gentleman) and motherly concern for the patient. Nursing came 'naturally' to women, second only to motherhood. Nightingale was certain enough of this to resist the suggestion that nursing should be controlled by examinations and registration, claiming that nurses could not be subject to this kind of test of their ability any more than mothers.

Medicine and nursing came to be seen as complementary activities in the sense that if nursing was feminine, medicine was masculine: the nurse was the ideal woman, the doctor the ideal man. His intelligent, active, pragmatic qualities were appropriate for curing and for the aggressive treatment of disease but not compatible with caring. One legacy of this traditional division of labour in which nurses carry out the decisions made by doctors is the lack of autonomy nurses currently experience as a group (Tschudin 1985/6).

Men in nursing

If nursing has been so strongly associated with the feminine, what does this suggest about men in nursing? Do men enter nursing because they wish to express the more 'feminine' aspects of their personality, as some have suggested? And if so, why do we find so many male nurses away from the bedside and in the top jobs? To answer these questions it is necessary to look at both the history of men in nursing and current theoretical trends within nursing ideology.

The history of men in nursing

In England and Wales at the turn of the century there were approximately 5700 men employed in nursing (Edwards 1984), of whom the majority worked in mental institutions. Here the custodial nature of the job—emphasised above any element of care—together with the potential need for strength in the restraint of violent patients, was compatible with current definitions of masculinity.

The situation was very different for the few men in general nursing; they were considered 'less than men'. There was no drive to recruit male general nurses but this may well have been less to do with their dubious gender status than the threat they represented to the status quo existing between nursing and medicine. Austin (1977) points out that any large-scale entry of men into general nursing might have unsettled the subordinate relationship of nursing to medicine, a relationship actually endorsed by nursing's female workforce and medicine's male one. However, the situation changed after the First World War, when with unemployment high, more or less any job became acceptable and there was an influx of men into nursing. The relationship between male asylum attendants and general nurses changed. Asylum attendants were regarded as inferior to general nurses as they came from a different and less privileged social and educational background, and their work was less prestigious because it was not as strongly identified as general nursing with the medical model.

The stigma associated with men in general nursing however remained, reflected in the allocation of male nurses to a separate part of the Register when registration was introduced in 1919. It was not until after the Second World War that training schools reduced their discrimination against male candidates and in 1949 there was sufficient recognition of male nurses for the male and female Registers to be combined. The Royal College of Nursing did not admit men until 1960. Since the Second World War many men have come into nursing as a result of doing similar work in the armed forces. In a study of 157 nurses by Rosen and Jones (1972), it was found that one third of the eighty-eight men studied had thought of nursing whilst in the forces. As one respondent said, a male nurse in the Army is doing a man's job; nobody thinks anything of it. Presumably there were few men in a position to think it strange as most men in the forces had to carry out such supposedly 'feminine' tasks as cooking, cleaning and mending.

Rosen and Jones found that, in general, male nurses were older, more likely to have previous work experience and to be married than female nurses of the same grade. Significantly, male nurses were far less likely to have come from a professional or middle-class background, or to have the same level of education as female nurses. Moreover, more men stayed on in nursing and wanted promotion. The study implies that—at least in the early 1970s— men found opportunities open to them in nursing that would otherwise have been denied them on the basis of class or educational achievement. It also suggests that men and women entered nursing for different reasons, that marginally more women went into nursing because of an interest in the work itself. More female than male recruits stated that interest in the personal relationships involved in the work were a significant factor; men seemed more attracted by the security the job seemed to offer.

Salvage (1985) notes that in 1980 almost half of the most senior nursing positions in management, education, the various professional organisations, trade unions and statutory bodies concerned with nursing were occupied by men, although in nursing as a whole, men constituted only approximately 10 per cent of the workforce. As Nuttall (1983) points out, the predominance of male nurses in senior posts in relation to their overall numbers does not mean that men are inherently more ambitious and more suitable for managerial jobs. It should be remembered, for example, that there are an increasing number of married women within nursing, yet it is still widely accepted that a woman will follow her husband to a new area should he be promoted and not *vice versa*: a female spouses's career aspirations are generally seen as secondary to those of her husband. It is expected that women (married or unmarried) will assume responsibility for ageing and other dependent relatives in a way not expected of men. There are then external reasons to help explain the disproportionate numbers of men in senior nursing posts.

There are also internal reasons. Women with children, for example, may face discrimination when applying for nursing jobs (see *Nursing Times* 1985: 'News'). In addition it has to be said that some female nurses appear to promote a hierarchical relationship between men and women within nursing. For example, one male nurse claims in a letter to the nursing press:

'Nursing is dominated by men in senior positions, not because men are better leaders, or aggressively climb to the top of the heap, but because female nurses would seem to prefer it that way. The 10 per cent of men are propelled upwards by the 90 per cent of women.' (Jones 1985)

All the nurses I spoke to were aware that male nurses were treated differently during training, both in School and in the clinical field. They could evade much of the discipline imposed on female trainees and could be more casual about observing hierarchical distinctions. They were often credited with having skills and knowledge beyond their level of training. Once qualified, male nurses were deferred to by nurses in training more than were female qualified staff of the same grade or experience. This, of course, is unsurprising if different attitudes towards male and female nurses can be observed among more senior staff.

Such discrimination raises a number of points. First there is the risk that, on the basis of a judgement distorted by prejudice about gender, male nurses will be given more responsibility than they can actually cope with. Second, there is a clear need for women within nursing to reject the conditioning they have received over the years about gender and to acknowledge their own worth and ability. Third, to integrate men into nursing on equal terms with women involves more than the striving of individual nurses to overcome the socialisation of gender role. Perhaps more than anything, it requires a rethinking of the beliefs which underlie much nursing theory, in which nursing autonomy and professionalisation have become associated with masculinity.

Masculinity and nursing theory

Men's relatively powerful position within nursing is not just the result of women's domestic responsibilities or even a simple reproduction of the social world outside. According to Austin (1977) there has been a deliberate attempt to introduce 'masculinity' into nursing at a fundamental level—that is, within the very knowledge base of nursing—as part of an attempt to establish nursing as a profession parallel to, rather than subordinate to, medicine.

Rational thought is not confined to the male brain. Yet there is a tradition within Western philosophy in which 'reason' is in some sense masculine, so that, by implication, women are less rational and more emotional than men. Nursing has in recent years tended to identify with this belief. According to Austin, this is demonstrated, for example, by the Salmon Report (1966) which questioned the ability of female nurses to act as managers. And there is an emphasis on the necessity for nursing practice to be based on the observable, the measurable and indeed the rational, despite the significance of the emotional and non-measurable aspects of the process of nursing. Rationality is unquestioningly accepted as the appropriate basis for nursing and it is men who are thought to bring this rational approach. The argument is not so much that male nurses are less emotional than their female counterparts or that the new, quantitatively derived knowledge is *inherently* masculine, but that men are in some way better equipped to deal with this knowledge (see, for example, Dingwall 1979).

The motives for this shift towards masculine values would appear to be, on the one hand, improved patient care, and on the other, to distinguish nursing as an entity separate from but equal to medicine. To do this, nurse theorists are attempting to identify those elements of a nurse's work which are specific to nursing, such as the nurse's involvement with the patient's activities of living. Henderson, for example, says

> 'The *unique* function of the nurse is to assist the individual, sick or well, in the performance of those activities contributing to health or its recovery (or to a peaceful death) that he would perform unaided if he had the necessary strength, will or knowledge and to do this in such a way as to help him gain independence as rapidly as possible.' (1966:15) (my emphasis)

However, the methods used to determine what this assistance should involve are essentially the same as those used by medicine to establish or justify its own knowledge base. As a result of adopting these methods, nursing enquiry proceeds predominantly through quantitative research such as statistical analysis. It resorts to what is essentially a fragmentary approach to understand something (the patient) it claims to perceive as a whole entity and more than the sum of its parts. In other words, nursing mimics important aspects of medicine in order to improve its standing but, paradoxically, claims by doing so to have shifted away from a medical model.

All this does not mean that quantitative methods of research are without value or that there is no place for men in nursing! There is no need to throw out the baby with the bathwater and we should beware efforts simply to invert the current trends within nursing. For example, in an attempt to redress the present imbalance, some go so far as to suggest that instead of adopting an approach informed by 'masculine' perspectives (that is, experience gained through specifically male gender socialisation) we should return to 'feminine' values. Oakley (1984), for example, suggests that the gender division of labour in health care which assumes the masculinity of doctors and the femininity of nurses has been one of the biggest problems for nurses—but also allows them their biggest opportunity. The emotional support associated with women in general and nurses in particular is, by and large, the outcome of social conditioning but it is nonetheless a valuable quality. Caring becomes an unashamedly feminine quality and the emphasis on caring within nursing becomes one of its strengths.

Unfortunately, the issue is not as straightforward as this. For one thing, regardless of the trends within nursing, it has always been viewed from the outside as inherently feminine. Moreover nursing has suffered because of the low value placed on feminine qualities, as the effects of the Griffiths Report demonstrate. The Royal College of Nursing (RCN) has shown particular concern about the restructuring of the health services subsequent to Griffiths. Its anxiety does not stem primarily from the relatively few nurses appointed as general managers—although this by itself is a disturbing trend. The main problem is whether or not nurses will be accountable to a nurse manager and how they will be able to convey their particular perspective on health care to those with power.

The RCN is most anxious about what happens at the unit level as this is where management structures affect patient care on a day-to-day basis. Its research has shown that units such as large hospitals are increasingly managed without a Director of Nursing Services. This means that the most senior level of management requiring a nursing qualification is that of Ward Sister/Charge Nurse and that nurses must turn to staff without nursing qualifications (be they doctors, administrators, treasurers or ex-members of the Armed Forces) for many decisions about day-to-day management such as staffing levels or equipment needs (RCN 1986a). The underlying aim of the Griffiths Report was to introduce a 'managerial culture' into the NHS (Evans 1983), to run the health services in accordance with market forces and economic considerations. Griffiths was about *rationalising* the NHS. As we have seen, rationality is perceived as a masculine quality, while nursing is understood to be feminine. This implicit value system has played some part in the latest restructuring of the NHS in which most of the senior nurses have been removed from managerial posts and as a result, the position of nurses in the NHS power structure has been threatened. We therefore cannot rest content with the identification of nursing with feminine qualities.

There are several variations of the argument in which nurses and nursing are understood in the light of ideal gender attributes. Some of these really seem to have gone over the top. Tschudin, for example, argues that nursing should exploit the gender division between its masculine and feminine elements and aim for a balance, rather like the Chinese principles of yin and yang which complement each other to form a whole. 'Feminine' qualities such as compassion and caring are balanced by 'masculine' ones of courage and leadership to bring about a balance within the process of nursing. Moreover,

> 'Male nurses in . . . their predictable male role are leading the female nurses by pointing out again the feminine values of nursing. They are attempting to give to the women the gift of themselves, their femininity. In accepting this gift wholly as it is meant, female nurses can give to the men in their ranks their true identity of maleness.' (1985/6:22)

This seems to suggest that masculine and feminine qualities are inevitably identified with men and women respectively.

Up to a point these arguments have been necessary because of the negative way in which qualities traditionally attributed to women have been valued, but the problem is that they lose sight of the fact that masculine and feminine qualities are *not* inherent in men and women but are largely the product of social conditioning. There is no built-in reason why, for example, women should be better at caring and men better at leading. We should therefore be attempting not to balance supposedly masculine and feminine qualities, but to challenge the assumption that particular qualities *are* predominantly masculine or feminine. Moreover, if nursing is to become an autonomous activity with its own unique body of knowledge, it must have the courage to find methods of research and analysis suited to its own needs, rather than unthinkingly accepting those more appropriate to other disciplines.

6

Challenging nurse stereotypes

In Chapter 5 we saw that sexuality and gender are evident within the very structure of nursing: nursing is female-dominated but values so-called 'masculine' qualities. Gender and sexuality also play a part in the way nurses are seen, both within and outside nursing. Gender expectations, including assumptions about sexual behaviour, help to construct present-day images and attitudes towards nurses, often with detrimental effects for the scope of nursing and the nurse–patient relationship. This chapter examines these images and looks at some of the reasons why they have developed. It discusses the effects of uniform, the concept of the nurse as a parental figure, and the association of nurses with service and submissiveness. Finally, it examines why it is important for these images of nurses to be challenged.

Images of female nurses

The images of female nurses fall into three main stereotypes: the angel/madonna (alias handmaiden), the battleaxe bitch and the sex-object/whore (Muff 1982; Salvage 1985). These images may be cross-cut by others, such as racial stereotypes. Black nurses suffer additionally from the way in which the sexuality of black women has become stereotyped, stemming historically from their sexual exploitation by white male colonialists (Benn 1985).

While the sources of stereotypes are predominantly outside nursing—for example, television, magazines, newspapers and novels—their impact on nurses, other health workers and patients

should not be underestimated. These images need to be challenged, but to do this successfully we must understand something
of the context in which they occur. Kalisch and her colleagues
(1983) studied the images of female nurses on American television
from the end of the Second World War until the 1970s and examined the way in which these images are linked to contemporary
social values. They found the value given to women's work in
general largely reflected in the television image of the nurse. The
authors show that in the 1950s, when the importance of women's
role as mother was stressed, nurses were not portrayed as technically skilled workers but as mother figures whose qualities were
those of the 'traditionally womanly treasure house of virtue'.
Good nurses were intuitive, self-effacing, self-sacrificing and comforting. There was certainly nothing to suggest that nurses were
objects of sexual interest. Generally speaking, the television nurse
in this era acted as 'Girl Friday' or handmaiden to the physician,
often to the point of devoting an entire 'career' to the quirks and
comforts of an individual doctor. Nursing was presented as an
inborn trait, a useful outlet for frustrated maternal feelings,
especially for those who did not marry.

The 1960s were years in which a woman's true place was in the
home, although little value was attached to the work she did
there. For the television nurse, according to Kalisch, this was the
era of the nurse as nonentity. In the two television classics of the
time (*Ben Casey* and *Doctor Kildare*), doctors were portrayed as
altruistic and non-materialistic, pledged to fighting injustice and
saving lives, while nurses were shown as carriers of clip-boards
and people who answered telephones. They were no more than
background characters.

This trend continued in the 1970s with one important
difference—the introduction of nurse characters solely to provide
sexual interest. The major exceptions to this pattern were the later
episodes of the long-running series M*A*S*H. Initially this programme treated nurses in a highly objectionable way, with, for
example, the sexual favours of the nurses being raffled off by the
doctors to raise money. However, in time and in accord with
changes in the image of American women in general, the portrayal of nurses changed. By the end of the series they are shown as
indispensable, independent, skilled and thoughtful, working in
equal partnership with other members of the health team.

Salvage (1982, 1985) has looked at media representations of

nurses in this country and sees a similar pattern. She finds the 'Carry On' and Richard Gordon films (such as *Doctor in the House*) redolent with stereotypical images of nurses as battleaxe (for example, Hattie Jacques) or sex object (Barbara Windsor). As in American portrayals, the actual work of nurses and the extent of their responsibilities are not represented. More recent television series such as *Only when I Laugh* and *Angels*—although not wildly popular with nurses themselves—did give a more realistic portrayal of nursing. However, much fiction, such as the doctor-nurse romances published by Mills & Boon, continues to perpetuate and exploit the stereotypes.

According to Kalisch and her co-writers, it is only in the past 10 to 15 years that nurses have been depicted as sex objects in television programmes and they believe that this trend represents a negative response to the demands and gains of the women's movement in these years. They argue that the idea of women determining their own lives prompted an insistence on the subordination of female characters by the handful of male writers responsible for these programmes. If this is the case it means that nurses cannot sit back and hope that wider social changes benefiting women in general will automatically improve the image of female nurses. Nurses themselves must take responsibility for challenging nurse stereotypes wherever they occur.

Images of male nurses

There are at least two images of the male nurse, both constructed around his sexuality. They are also linked to the norms concerning the sexual division of labour in which nursing is regarded as a woman's occupation. It is doubtful, though, whether one of these images is a genuine stereotype. This is the caricature of the male nurse as a Casanova, supposedly based on the fact that male nurses have chosen an occupation in which they will be surrounded by women. As one male nurse said: 'It is always assumed by patients that I'm chasing after one or other of the young nurses. They want to know who wears the sexiest underwear.' But this image of the male nurse does not appear to be widely held. In fact it was only suggested to me by male nurses on the strength of what patients had said to them. This may mean that it is not an actual stereotype but part of the individual nurse-patient relationship, and something of a strategy for coping with the implications of the *predominant* image of the male nurse in which it is assumed he is homosexual.

The 'logic' underlying the association between male nurses and homosexuality is as follows: the man who enters nursing has failed to make his way in a man's world and now only a female world is available to him. He is further emasculated by taking on 'women's work' in which he is expected to demonstrate 'feminine' qualities such as caring and gentleness and in which, at least to begin with, he will be subordinate to women. And if his masculinity is in question, so too is his sexuality. It has been shown earlier how masculinity can be shored up in our culture by an aggressive genital sexuality; there is an assumed link between the two, so that anything which seems to affect one also implicates the other. This view of male nurses mistakenly sees a correlation between gender role and sexual preference.

Male nurses are not exclusively heterosexual. But a proportion of female nurses are lesbian without this becoming the predominant stereotype. Regardless of the number of male nurses who are homosexual the stereotype of the male nurse, like those of female nurses, needs to be challenged because of the way it may interfere with the process of nursing.

The development of stereotypes

We have seen that both male and female nurses are regarded as objects of sexual curiosity. Moreover, while it is not uncommon for women in general to be sexually objectified, there is something specific and more thoroughgoing about the way in which women-as-nurses are treated. The stereotypes of nurses are probably so powerful and well-defined for a number of reasons.

We have already seen how nursing has been female-dominated, and how it corresponds with what is seen as appropriate work for women in our culture's division of labour. One result of the identification of nursing with women has been for the public to see nursing as the embodiment of feminine values, with nurses as self-sacrificing, submissive and exploitable in the service of doctors and patients. Yet nurses are not without power: they are often seen as analogous to the mother figure who can be both tender and terrible. Simultaneous fantasy and horror can be prompted in some by helplessness and passivity. Men, according to gender-role expectations, are not allowed to be helpless and passive, yet they are rendered so when they become patients. At one level this helplessness can be frightening, especially when it makes them dependent on women, but at another level it provides some sort of sexual charge (see, for example Fagin and Diers (1984), who see nursing as a metaphor not only for motherhood but also for intimacy and sex). The female nurse therefore comes to represent a focus for the male patient's mixed feelings. The same helplessness and dependency must have different, but possibly just as powerful implications for the relationship between male patients and male nurses, female patients and male nurses, and female patients and female nurses. Finally within this context, the fact that the nurse is de-personalised through the wearing of uniform is also significant.

The next part of this chapter looks at all these issues: the role of uniform, nurses as parental figures and the association of nurses with service and submission as important factors in the development of nurse stereotypes, and examines how they can be challenged.

Uniform

Uniform is 'the dress worn by members of the same body'. More tellingly, the adjective 'to be uniform' means to be 'unchanging in form or character' or 'conforming to the same standard or rule'. There is a sense, then, that by wearing a standard mode of dress, individuals can be labelled as one of a kind: the wearer of a uniform becomes a blank slate on to which an identity can be projected from the outside.

Olesen and Whittaker (1968), in their dissection of the traditional nursing uniform, describe how it conceals the female form as far as possible. The starched bib of the apron, for example, attempts to disguise the presence of the nurse's breasts; starched collar and cuffs add masculine, militaristic touches; even black or white stockings, they claim, serve to remind the observer that this is a person in uniform who should be regarded as asexual.

According to Strauss, like earlier nurses, 'the present-day one has a strong shoulder for the patient to rest his troubles upon but, metaphorically speaking, her very bosom is absent as an object for him to gaze upon!' (1966:90). The implication is that the good nurse is not seductive. Not everyone would agree with Strauss. A group of nurses in the United States, supposedly distressed by the way in which nurses were portrayed on television as 'plain, middle-aged and rather custodial-looking', took action by volunteering for a pictorial feature in *Playboy* in 1983. In this they appeared first in their uniforms, performing various nursing duties, and then off-duty, without their uniforms or in fact any other clothing. Unfortunately they protested against one image of the nurse by reinforcing another.

Many people seem to be only too aware of the nurse as a sexual object. Evidence of this can be gleaned from the titles of many pornographic films (*Private Nurse*, *Student Nurse*, etc.), from cartoons, get-well cards and so on, as Salvage points out (1982). The role of uniform in this is hard to place, although other women who wear uniform, such as waitresses or even schoolgirls, are also the subjects of pornography. Perhaps the 'turn-on' associated with uniform is because it has no relation to the individual who wears it, but is instead associated with the role of the wearer. In the case of nurses, their role as servant and/or mother is associated with the characteristics of submissiveness *and* authoritarianism, both of which can be eroticised.

As suggested earlier, uniform can reduce an individual to a mere cut-out figure on which observers can project whatever they desire. It has been observed that all nursing uniforms have their share of white, and acccording to Kreuger (1978), the ideology of nursing links all sorts of moral qualities to the meaning of white—the clean life, purity, endless obedience and a quasi-religious sense of service to the sick. But it would seem that it is simultaneously the very suggestion of purity and service that makes nurses (and nuns, too) the subject of sexual fantasies. Boerigger, for example, says of the effect of nursing uniform: 'man is piqued by the quirk of wanting to possess and conquer that which is unobtainable or virginally untouched, and hence pure' (1973). Muff (ibid) has noted that many male observers have an interest in believing that the female nurse attempts to obscure her 'femininity' by her uniform and demeanour, but is unsuccessful and instead surrounds herself with an aura of sexuality. But Muff raises the question of whose sexuality this is. She suggests it is not always the nurse's. What should be guarded against is the idea that men know women's desires better than women do themselves (a dangerous argument, also commonly used to 'explain' rape). As Muff points out, what the observer sees is merely a reflection of

his own desire, which he then defends by claiming that it origin-
ates with women.

Some of the female nurses I spoke to felt drained of their own
personality when they wore uniform and conscious of an alien
sexual identity that was pinned on them by observers. However, it
has to be said that many nurses enjoy wearing uniform, especially
in its more traditional forms. For example, in a competition in the
nursing press to create a new uniform for the 1980s, the winning
costume was specially designed to 're-introduce femininity while
maintaining professionalism' (*Nursing Times*: 1980). It won
because it took the cuffs, belt, linen cap and apron of the traditional uniform that nurses were thought to hanker after and
brought them 'up to date'. One of the reasons why nurses want to
retain the various accessories of traditional regalia is that they are
often used to indicate the wearer's status. One of the Mills & Boon
authors is sufficiently in touch with the realities of nursing to
write:

> 'Brenda ... rose to her feet, smoothing down the well-cut
> uniform dress in the dark green fabric that was still a jealously
> guarded right of the senior staff of the Princess Beatrice ... The
> juniors wore the new regulation clothes but longed for the
> privilege of wearing the dignified and graceful dresses and caps
> supplied when they reached the dizzy heights of staff nurse and
> beyond.' (Cooper 1985:16–17)

Certainly, many of the nurses I interviewed felt strongly about
a change from traditional to national uniform. Some were largely
drawn into nursing by the uniform, although they were unable to
explain why. These same nurses however recognised that they had
a highly romantic view of nursing before they began training.

Men and uniform

The male nurse's uniform does not convey the same messages as
the female nurse's uniform, and ultimately plays little role in con-
structing a stereotype of the male nurse. Generally speaking, a
male nurse wears either a white coat over 'mufti' or a short white
jacket with dark trousers. He is frequently confused with doctors,
radiographers, technicians and other male health workers who
might also wear some sort of uniform. Significantly, most of the
male nurses I spoke to said that patients very often assume that

they belong to an occupational group with higher status than nurses (such as doctors)—simply because they are men. Doctors had little idea of who or what these men were. This was particularly the experience of junior nurses. However, while the male nurse's uniform does not clearly indicate his role, it does endorse certain aspects of his image, if more by way of omission than anything else. The uniform does not attempt to disguise the physical shape of its wearer. Indeed it could be argued that the 'dentist jacket' worn by many male nurses does the reverse, accentuating the width of the shoulders. The purity symbolised by the wearing of white, and its connotations of virginity do not apply to men in the same way, or prompt the ambivalent response that they do with women. It is not just that our double-standard society places little value on virginity in men, but also that men's virginity actually has a *negative* value; it is seen as a peculiar state and one which again questions masculinity. Moreover, the wearing of white by men is obviously offset by other considerations, such as status. Male doctors have been wearing white coats for decades without compromising their masculinity and while male nurses do not have the same status as doctors, it seems there is sufficient analogy for the wearing of white to have little serious implication for their image.

This is reflected in the way that male nurses feel about their uniform. The male nurses I spoke to experienced a mixture of initial pride *and* feelings of awkwardness at the beginning of their training but with time these feelings gave way to a more *laissez-faire* attitude. 'We felt like wallies for a few weeks in these dentist's jackets, but they *are* practical' (Staff nurse). The various impractical accessories of the female uniform, such as caps, cuffs and frills are adapted from the dress of the nineteenth-century maid and help to remind us of the servitude expected of nurses. Significantly the male uniform is devoid of such embellishment. The authority inspired by uniform is unopposed by frills and other feminine symbols denoting servitude. As one male student nurse remarked, 'A uniform's a uniform. It gives you that air of being detached and lets you get in close because you can say "Come on, I'm a nurse; don't give me this."'

Uniform: to be or not to be

Uniform would seem to play a significant role in maintaining stereotypes—at least of the female nurse. Szasz (1982) has gone so far as to describe the wearing of uniform as 'unprofessional' because it serves as a reminder of the unthinking obedience and servitude traditionally expected of nurses. She also sees uniform as imposing a distance between the nurse and patient and actually reducing communication rather than enhancing it. She also doubts that uniform allows a sense of group identity, pointing out that, as attempts at industrial action have shown, there is little co-hesion or unity amongst nurses. Nursing is fragmented, not least by its hierarchy, which is often made evident through uniform. We must therefore ask, is uniform really necessary?

It is difficult to dispense with the idea of uniform altogether. Among its other virtues, it protects nurses' own clothes, provides a sense—albeit limited—of group identity, saves the nurse money on clothes and—where laundry services are still in existence—can save the nurse a lot of washing and ironing. Uniform does not always demonstrate the occupation of the wearer and clearly does not provide a 'Who's Who' for the patient—which is often a plea in its defence. But as one nurse said:

> 'I think that we've taught patients about uniform and therefore patients expect uniform. I don't think we'll ever abolish uniform in general nursing so what we've got to do is offer a *range* of uniform. First of all we've got to put everyone in the same colour—it doesn't matter what level they are; the person running the ward should know what qualifications they've got—but then offer nurses a range of uniforms and let them choose which type suits their personality.'

Alternatively, any clothing that is functional and of a certain pre-scribed colour which identifies the nurse as a nurse could be con-sidered, although one disadvantage of this is that nurses would lose laundry facilities and would have to fight for a uniform allow-ance to cover the cost of providing their own clothes. Such a move away from the present system would also be unpopular among many nurses who seem very attached to the traditional uniform.

It is possible that it is nurses in training who are most attached to traditional uniform because of its use in marking hierarchy. Hierarchy is undoubtedly important to many trained nurses but additionally, when you are right at the bottom of the pile, any-thing that signifies that you are moving up has special meaning. Also, very junior nurses, because of their lack of experience, *want* to be identifiable as such, so that people do not make demands on them that they cannot fulfil. But once a nurse is confident in her work it is easier for her to recognise that proficiency comes from within, rather from anything that a uniform suggests. The solution would seem to be for qualified nurses to choose a uniform of standard colour from a range of styles, which readily distinguishes them from nurses in training. However, this is only a partial solution to the problem of uniform.

More importantly, whether it is called self-knowledge or navel-gazing, nurses need the opportunity to examine their personal attitudes towards uniform and what it represents for them. This may lead to a deeper understanding of their relationships with other nurses, other health workers, and patients. In addition, given the way in which patients are stripped of their own clothing in hospital, the opportunity to discuss the meaning uniform holds for individual nurses may be useful not only for their own development but also to bring insight into the experience of the patient.

Nurses as parental figures

Another factor influencing images of nurses concerns people's attitudes to dependency, and the strange mixture of emotions it may provoke. Responses to dependency in adulthood appear to vary between men and women and can perhaps be traced to early experiences with parents. Significantly, an analogy has been drawn between the nuclear family and the health-care setting, in which the nurse plays the part of mother, the doctor is the father and the patient is their child (see for example Oakley 1984; McCurdy 1982).

The association of female nurses with mothers is particularly well recognised. Susannah Wright (1985), speaking as a patient, makes an explicit link. First of all, she argues, the nurse carries out certain tasks fulfilled by a mother—washing, feeding, dosing, instructing and putting her charges to bed (although it has to be said these tasks could equally be carried out by a father). Wright suggests that the adult retains or incorporates some of the characteristics of a child, such as the need for nurturance. With time, she argues, we all become our own mothers as best we can. But various crises such as illness or hospitalisation reduce our effectiveness in mothering ourselves, and as patients we temporarily regress to being a needy child again. Wright suggests nurses are in a position to nurture and comfort us in this crisis, at both an emotional and a physical level. Other writers go further. Newton, for example, suggests 'the first job of the nurse is to be a mother surrogate' (1981:351). Despite the cosiness suggested by the analogy between mothers and nurses, it should be remembered that many men's and women's relationships with their mothers are far from straightforward. There have been numerous attempts to explain the mixed feelings people have towards their mothers and how such ambivalence can be extended to women in general. Easlea (1981), for example, suggests this conflict of emotions arises for all men in male-dominated societies because of the way in which masculine gender identity develops. Obviously men are born of women, and as infants they are usually suckled and cared for by women. Infants, say Easlea, come to see their mother's body as an extension of their own, and yet boys in particular must end this identification with the mother and become separate if they are to become men. Most adults at some point in their lives want to recreate the sense of wholeness and closeness associated with early childhood, but for men to do so arouses a particular ambivalence. To re-merge with the mother-figure threatens their masculine identity. To add to their confusion, men have been socialised into believing themselves superior to women. As men, they are expected to penetrate and impregnate the women who paradoxically represent both their inferiors and the person who brought them into the world.

This suggests that if an analogy between the female nurse and the mother holds any meaning, we should expect the male patient to experience a degree of ambivalence towards the female nurse. She not only represents a member of the 'second' (that is, subordinated) sex who happens to wield considerable power over him, but also a figure on whom any dependency deeply threatens his masculine identity. In general little attention has been given to women's views of other women as mother figures. Eichenbaum and Orbach (1983) provide one exception. They state how understandings of masculinity and femininity are learned initially through the mother as principal nurturer. Mothers therfore play a central role in creating the psychologies of women as well as men. Not only do Eichenbaum and Orbach see the mother/daughter relationship as the main arena in which female gender role is forged, but they also consider that it forms a model for future relationships with other women. The mother unconsciously restrains herself from meeting her daughter's childhood needs as often as she might because this would create an unfair expectation for the daughter that her needs will be met by others later in life. The mother therfore appears inconsistent in her support of the daughter and their relationship becomes ambivalent. This ambivalence is then projected by the daughter on to women in general; they may experience in their relationships with other women (including nurses) the buried resentment which has been directed against the mother. Both men and women therefore may have mixed feelings towards the mother figure and perhaps towards women as a group. From this comes the view of women as having a dual character, symbolising both good and bad.

If Oakley and others are right, that the nurse is a mother figure and the doctor a father figure, where does the male nurse fit in? Patients' attitudes towards male and female nurses can vary a great deal because of the difference in gender-role expectations. This may mean that male and female nurses will fulfil different roles until such time as gender roles in our society come to overlap more closely. It cannot be assumed, however, that the male nurse represents a father figure. To begin with, in the context of our cultural assumptions and attitudes towards fatherhood, the concept of the male nurse as father figure sits uneasily with the stereotype of the male nurse as homosexual. Second, it is not, as yet, widely acceptable for fathers in our society to be involved in nurturing children. Instead father figures are primarily and unambiguously associated with power and authority. As a result, if male nurses *should* in some way represent father figures for patients, it would have far-reaching and negative implications for their role. It would, for example, undermine their ability to act as the patient's advocate, because of the imbalance of power between nurse and patient. However, while not necessarily representing father figures, male nurses are more clearly associated with power than female nurses—a point I shall return to later (see pp. 91–94).

The nurse as mother: implications

Seeing the nurse-patient relationship in terms of a parent–child relationship, and using psychoanalytic theory to analyse this may give some insight into the different expectations male and female patients have of nurses, and the way in which some images of the nurse are constructed, while an understanding of the complexities of the parent-child relationship may provide some explanation for the way many nurses see themselves. For example, female nurses' identification with a mother figure may partly explain their traditional lack of political assertiveness: the analogy between female nurses and mothers rests in part on the way in which both are seen as selfless and all-giving.

As the image of female nurses as mothers seems to come as much from within nursing as from outside it, much can be done to change it by nurses themselves. The 'mother-earth' ethos can be found in the idea that nurses must be seen to cope in all circumstances, and the difficulty that nurses find in saying that they are over-stretched. This ethos is imposed to a certain extent on the nurse by the way in which nursing itself is organised. It is, for example, only very recently that senior nurses have become involved in any attempt to oppose cutbacks in NHS funding or rapid turnover in bed occupancy. By implication, they have expected nurses simply to work harder in order to provide the same standard of care as before the cuts. This situation will only really improve when senior nurses achieve a clear understanding of the day-to-day problems experienced by those working at the 'sharp end', through closer co-operation. Recognition should also be given to a similar ethos held by some individual nurses who enjoy seeing themselves as selfless and indispensable. They seem to want to be busy to the point of frenzy. As one nurse described it: 'The real buzz is to go home at the end of the day absolutely exhausted and unable to move saying "Gosh, I had ten, twelve patients to look after!"' Here is the earth-mother, caring for her charges against impossible odds. And yet the only care possible under these conditions is the fulfilment of tasks like bedbaths or mouth care. There can be no opportunity to draw up an overall profile of the patient's health needs, or any room for the patient to discuss anxieties. Sadly, many nurses seem to enjoy working in this frantic and fragmented way precisely because it allows them no space for these concerns. Approaching nursing as an obstacle race protects them from the patient's emotional needs. This defensive strategy has become necessary because, despite a growing expectation that the nurse will 'enter the patient's world', she is given inadequate training and support to allow her to cope with the emotional needs of patients should these be allowed to emerge.

Nurses, power and servitude

Closely linked to the phenomenon of nurses as parental figures are the issues of power, service and submission associated with the nurse-patient relationship and the doctor-nurse relationship. We have seen that women have been associated with nursing because of their ascribed gender role. Significantly, gender can be seen to be directly linked to the structures of prestige and power in any society (Ortner and Whitehead 1981). Power distribution in the health services is similar to the way in which power and privilege are distributed in society as a whole (Versluysen 1980). In our society, power is, in general, held by men. Women may have more influence in the domestic sphere but there are relatively few women in powerful public positions. Individual women may wield power over individual men but they rarely hold power direct. Nurses, though presently not a powerful group (as demonstrated by their low pay), do individually have a certain amount of power in relation to their patients and patients' relatives. In addition, some nurses are powerful within nursing: the hierarchy of nursing is more explicit than in most institutions. In this part of the chapter I will begin by looking at power relations in fiction between men and women in general and between nurses and patients and nurses and doctors, to help demonstrate the relationship between gender, sexuality and power. Although it can be argued that fiction exaggerates this relationship it is still a useful source of examples, as exaggeration may help to crystallise what generally occurs at a less perceptible level.

Power and women

Feminine gender is generally associated with passivity, but as Coward (1984) has said, in women's fantasies at least, passivity does not necessarily mean powerlessness. In romantic fiction written primarily for women by women, a happy ending (generally marriage) is important not only for moral reasons but also because of the transfer of power from a man to a woman that becomes evident once he admits some dependency and commitment.

Looking more specifically at fictional doctor/nurse romances, we frequently find that the metamorphosis of an arrogant doctor into a warm and needy person is triggered by an attractive woman who is also a 'damned good nurse'. As with general fiction, by the end of these hospital romances, although the doctor is still taking most of the decisions and the nurse is still questioning how she came to be so lucky, the balance of power has perceptibly shifted. The nurse is now the 'power behind the throne', secure in the knowledge that without her, 'her man' would be a shadow of his new-found self.

It is not uncommon in general fictional romance for gruff, tough men to be rendered helpless and dependent on the heroine through illness or injury. Such dependency allows the woman to acquire a measure of power (again similar to that of a mother over a child) while allowing the man the chance to recognise his need, or even his love for the heroine. Whether this sort of fiction is prompted by or actually shapes women's imaginations is debatable, but Coward thinks the literature suggests there is a positive quest for power in these fantasies.

Now does this have any significance for nurses? Certainly in fiction there is an idea of female nurses as sufficiently powerful to be in a position to search actively among their patients for a future husband, as the following passage suggests:

'She walked among them, borne on her Sister shoes, trailing mercy and libido, followed by the medicine trolley. "Aaahh," they sighed. "Ooohh," they groaned. Deeply they breathed in oxygen, demurely peed in bottles under bedclothes. "Which bed will it be?" thought Sister.' (Hoban 1976:10)

In this novel (*Kleinzeit*), not only are the patients sexually aware of the Sister but she is actively looking for someone in their midst who will meet her sexual and emotional need. Once asked by a doctor why she was looking for a sick man rather than a well one she could only shrug her shoulders. But it is difficult to think of many non-nursing situations which allow women the same power over adult men.

Many of the nurses I spoke to in the course of researching this book suggested that women enter nursing because of a need to be needed—and that to be needed is, to a certain extent, one way of being powerful. Williams (1978) has noted how conditions of helplessness and the tasks associated with it breach the normal relationship between women and men in our society. Washing, feeding, and other tasks generally performed by adults for themselves in varying degrees of privacy become processes which reduce the adult male to the status of a child when they are performed for him by a female. By seeing nursing as a vocation, according to Williams, the adult status of the patient is rescued by the knowledge that the nurse is doing these tasks for her own fulfilment. Yet clearly the nurse gains some power from this situation and, perhaps less clearly, this power is in turn resented by those who are accustomed to being in a more powerful position (notably, men).

At the same time, the line between nursing and servicing is a fine one, and the power of the person being serviced is considerable. To give a non-nursing example:

'She hated the thought of waiting on me in bed. She didn't do it for her husband and she couldn't see why she should do it for me. To take breakfast in bed was something I never did except at Woodruff's place. I did it expressly to annoy and humiliate her.' (Miller 1965)

Needless to say this hero's power is such that he also eventually has his hostess service him sexually, hinting at the link between power and sex.

Just as men can endorse power through sex, power held by women can be confiscated through sex. The portrayal of 'Big Nurse' in *One Flew Over the Cuckoo's Nest* shows, first of all, how a female nurse in a psychiatric hospital is distrusted by her patients largely because of the power she holds over them. As one patient describes it:

'I've watched her grow more skilful over the years. Practice has steadied and strengthened her until now she wields a sure power that extends in all directions, on hairlike wires too small for anybody's eye but mine; I see her sit in the centre of this web of wires like a watchful robot . . . know every second which wire runs where and just what current to send up to get the result she wants.' (Kesey 1973:27)

Assertive, independent or 'stroppy' women are frequently resented and, sure enough, Big Nurse gets her come-uppance when she is attacked by another patient. Significantly the attack has elements of a sexual assault.

'with terror forever ruining any other look she might ever try to use again, screaming when he grabbed for her and ripped her uniform all the way down the front, screaming again when the two nippled circles started from her chest and swelled out and out, bigger than anybody had ever imagined, warm and pink in the light ... doctors and supervisors and nurses prying those heavy red fingers out of the white flesh of her throat.' (*ibid*: 250)

Rendering Big Nurse half-naked—attacking some aspect of her sexual identity—was the surest way of permanently damaging her powerfulness; again we find that sexual identity and power are often closely interwoven.

It is not only the relationship between nurses and patients that can be seen in terms of power and sexual innuendo. The disparity of power between doctors and nurses provides the very basis of the 'thrill' in popular novels dealing with hospital romance. Take, for example, the Mills & Boon classic *Nurse Foster* by Rhona Uren. In this story a young Sister, perhaps over-proud of her status, is rapidly brought down to size by the equally status-conscious, handsome-if-cruel Doctor Theodore Smythe. He does this initially by speaking to her as if she were a student (!) and demanding that she address him as 'Sir', all the while staring at her with eyes full of anger, contempt and (of course) a certain *je ne sais quoi* that 'liquefied her bones'. This author implies that it is not only acceptable for a doctor to decide on appropriate behaviour for nurses but that to be treated with contempt is something of a turn-on. If this were not bad enough, our heroine later 'finds her body betraying her' and responding to his passionate kisses even though these seem yet another attempt to degrade her. Finally the 'hero' attempts to rape Nurse Foster—for the 'worthy' reason of preventing her from making the mistake of marrying someone else. When he finally declares his own love for her he 'explains' all his previous behaviour with the rationale 'Haven't you heard that a man always hurts the thing he loves?' Sadly with this, 'the knowledge came to her that whatever he decreed, whatever he said she must do, she would gladly obey.' This stress on humiliation and the threat of violence is an alarming trend which is increasingly found in general 'romantic' fiction written for women, very often by women. This genre of writing has been given the nickname of 'Bodice Rippers' by the publishing world because of its essential element: the heroine must have her clothes torn from her quivering flesh by a series of brutal men. What is perhaps worse, these women are depicted as somehow quite separate from their bodies, emerging remarkably unscathed from the most violent abuse and helpless against their own irrational desires. Unfortunately there are clear parallels between the Bodice Rippers and the Nurse Foster variety of doctor-nurse romance, although fiction concerned with hospital romance is generally seen as harmless entertainment.

Nurse Foster is not the standard nurse heroine. She is a bit uppity and is seen to need a strong hand. The more typical heroine of these romances is a member of the angel/madonna species, physically as well as spiritually blemish-free. For example, 'her pale skin was smooth and added to the Madonna calm of her lovely mouth.' (Cooper 1985:5)

Despite the Health Service's dependence on its black workers, the heroes and heroines of these romances are always white, although recently black nurses and doctors have been introduced as part of the supporting cast.

In doctor-nurse romances, nurses seem to spend their entire life on duty, although it is difficult to piece together what their work entails. In *The Happy Ward* (Cooper:*ibid*), the heroine, Sister Kaye Harcourt of the paediatric ward, is mostly depicted either as 'scooping up' crying infants into her arms, the children responding immediately to the softness of her breast and her huge trustworthy eyes, or servicing doctors: it is at this level that she seems to have most in common with other members of the nursing staff. Moreover, there is some strange connection between carrying out chores for doctors and sexual excitement. For example, 'He (Doctor Orson Latimer) saw Nurse Benson coming out of the ward kitchen. 'I hope you were putting on the kettle' he said. She blushed and laughed' (*ibid*:72).

According to Stein (1978) the traditional relationship between doctors and nurses (of dominance and subservience respectively) has gone largely unchallenged for decades. The rhetoric of nursing may suggest 'collaboration' between them, but reality is different. Admittedly nurses do exercise some control and make decisions concerning patient care, but they contrive to do this without appearing to detract from a doctor's authority. Stein calls this the 'doctor-nurse game'. The nurse who is successful at this game is, Stein argues, rewarded by being acknowledged as a good nurse. She who fails to play the game, however, risks unpopularity. Her competence is questioned and she may be described as a 'bitch' or a 'man-hater'. It is interesting that what at first sight appears to be an issue concerning the boundaries of role (medical versus nursing) is clearly experienced in terms of sexuality and gender. McFarlane, in her Marsden lecture on nursing images and reality (1985), could be referring to the doctor-nurse game when she states that while most doctors no longer see the nurse as an assistant in their work, this change has been accompanied by resentment and anger. And if the image of the nurse as hand-maiden has taken a pasting, it has not yet been replaced by one of the nurse as colleague. One reflection of this, and of the way in which many nurses collude with this process, is the number of lec-tures given to nurses by doctors, with no acknowledgement of the differences between the realities of medicine and of nursing. There has been an understanding that lectures given by doctors are in some way better than those given by nurses and that such lectures will invest nursing with some of medicine's prestige. *The Happy Ward* spells out the paternalism of this system. The hero, Doctor Latimer, when lecturing to nurses assures them 'I'll put it very simply'. And just in case they cannot work out the difference between facts and waffle he adds, when he feels it necessary, 'Now write this down and learn it'. Meanwhile the nurses look at him 'wide-eyed and impressed' (Cooper 1985). The incidence of doctors lecturing to nurses may have declined in recent years but this could well be because of shortfalls in nursing finances rather than through any change of attitude amongst nurse tutors.

While the representation of nurses in romantic fiction is in many ways far from reality, in 'real life' the concept of the nurse as colleague still seems remote, despite the partial acceptance by doctors of nurse practitioners, practice nurses and others. Signifi-cantly, pressure to extend the role of the nurse often comes from doctors themselves—where such an extension is in their best inter-est. For example, 'Junior doctors—tired of being dragged from their beds at night to administer to patients—have joined battle to extend the role of the nurse' (*Nursing Times* 1980 **76**:1245). Unfortunately, all that glitters is not gold; the extended role of the nurse can mean that they become responsible primarily to doctors rather than to other nurses, doing those tasks that doctors are weary of doing and moving further away from a concept of nurs-ing as an autonomous body of knowledge and practice.

Power and men

Perhaps by now it will come as no surprise that the position of male nurses *vis-à-vis* patients and doctors in terms of power relations and expectations of service is very different from that of female nurses—but not necessarily better. Groff (1984), in an article in the American nursing literature, writes how demeaning he finds the term 'male nurse', which suggests to him that he is a member of sub-species of nurses. Merely on the basis of his sex he is not the real thing. He experiences this primarily from his female colleagues but also in his first meetings with many of his patients; their initial response is frequently surprise, followed by regret. Regret comes from assumptions that with a male nurse to care for them, patients will miss out on being comforted and on some routine aspects of nursing care such as back rubs. As patients (male and female), they will not feel free to show their emotions and they will not receive the same kind of emotional support they would be given by a female nurse.

Underlying these assumptions is a particular image of men which has certain implications for male nurses. It is thought that purely because of their sex, male nurses have the power to dominate their patients, or to dismiss many of their needs. To think that men might *care* is rather like suggesting pigs might fly. Groff sees an analogy between the lengths male nurses must go to in order to be seen to be as caring as their female colleagues and the fact that female doctors have to be much brighter than the majority of male doctors in order to be recognised as intellectually equal. It is, says Groff, both degrading and rewarding when his patients discover 'with a sense of wonder' that he is a gentle person.

It is particularly interesting that Groff thought patients did not feel they would receive the expected level of emotional support from a male nurse. This suggests something about the power relations which may exist between male nurses and their patients, as people are reluctant to share their fears and emotions with those they experience as more powerful than themselves; it leaves them too vulnerable. The problem seems to be widespread despite the good intentions of male nurses. Of those I spoke to, several expressed frustration that they were not trusted by patients to provide emotional support. For example:

> 'There was one chap . . . I mean, I cried even if he wouldn't. His life just suddenly seemed to fall to pieces . . . and he just wouldn't cry. I kept saying "It's all right for you to cry," but he wouldn't. He allowed me to shave him before his operation but

I wasn't allowed to sit with him if he was upset. He'd say "Go away, I'll be all right in a minute". He was more open with the female nurses. He was more prepared to talk to them about his marriage and how things had gone wrong with that; it was just easier for him to be the weaker person in that situation. I suppose with me he was playing the male role—trying to be strong.'

Male patients seem to have a particular problem, that stems from the way in which they have been socialised into denying or hiding their feelings. To discuss their emotions, especially with another man, would be to cast doubt on their masculinity. Not surprisingly, the relationship between male patients and male nurses is often uneasy, as this nurse's comment indicates:

'I think male patients would get quite embarrassed if they got close to me. And they never used to know how to say goodbye. They'd give a box of chocolates and a kiss to the female nurses—but how do you say goodbye to a male nurse?'

The nurse's gender can therefore cross-cut either his or her personal characteristics and intentions or those of the patient. While, for example, the male student quoted earlier was prepared to disregard considerations of masculinity and cry, the patient would not. Perhaps this is not surprising given the dependence of the patient; he is already vulnerable without risking his gender identity. What is interesting is that despite his relative powerlessness, the patient in this account manages to retain some control of the situation—even if it is only to ask the nurse to leave him alone for a while or to choose who he *will* unburden himself to. A female patient would be in a different position in relation to a male nurse and, as the following example suggests, may feel it necessary to use a female nurse as mediator. As one male student nurse told me: 'One lady complained. I wish she had said it to me actually; it would have been a lot better. She said "I don't like him giving me bedpans". I don't know why she didn't say it to me.'

In terms of male nurses' relationships with doctors, we have to do without the insight offered by romantic fiction as, to my knowledge, it has not yet taken a male nurse as its hero. This is in itself significant. Perhaps the absence of the male nurse as romantic hero can be partly explained by the stereotype of the male nurse as homosexual and this type of fiction does not yet extend to gay romance. It should be remembered that the principal readership of doctor-nurse romance is female. It appears that for this audience the thrill of romance is best achieved by a scenario in which a powerless female nurse profoundly affects an obviously powerful figure—the doctor. The absence of male nurses is therefore a comment on the power held by male nurses; there is insufficient disparity in power between male and female nurses to make for any kind of sexual thrill. Presumably readers would find romances between female doctors and male nurses disappointing for similar reasons.

In the absence of any insight offered directly by fiction, let us turn to the words of male nurses themselves. Some told me of what can only be called blind prejudice towards them from male doctors. As one charge nurse said: 'Some doctors found it a bit odd— a male nurse. I did obstetrics for eight weeks and one of the three gynaecologists thought it was most peculiar, this man being there. And he was a man himself!'. Male doctors, like male patients, seem uneasy about how they should relate to male nurses, especially where factors such as age do not clarify the authority of the doctor. Male nurses I spoke to had observed that the young male doctors who clearly had no difficulty making demands of female nurses, avoided working with male nurses. This implies that the doctor-nurse relationship (or that aspect of it in which nurses service the needs of the doctor) remains heavily dependent on the feminine identity of nursing.

Not only do male nurses fail to fit the handmaiden role, but the confidence or assertiveness provided by their gender training also means that their relationships with doctors are qualitatively different from those of female nurses. The latter are often self-effacing in the presence of doctors, even if they are older, or have the benefit of a non-nursing degree or broad work experience prior to nursing. Male nurses are not only less self-effacing, but also more prepared to challenge doctors over patient care. Although Stein (*ibid*) does not examine the extent to which male nurses become involved in the 'doctor-nurse game', male nurses would probably get a lower score than female nurses. Yet while the assertive female nurse is seen as a 'man hater' because she does not comply with the rules, it is unlikely the relative assertiveness of the male nurse will be attributed to 'deviant' sexuality.

Patient power

Within the nurse-patient relationship both male and female nurses can become figures of considerable power and this needs to be recognised, particularly in any move towards developing nursing as a form of patient advocacy. Of course, the power dynamic varies tremendously according to the different personalities involved as well as the sexes. While nurses should recognise the power they can exert over patients, there must also be some awareness that the situation can be reversed. The personal services offered by nurses, for example, can be used to demonstrate the distribution of power between nurse and patient and can be exploited by *either* party. Later on (pp. 99–101, 104–106) it will be argued that embarrassment can be seen as an indication of the locus of this power and, significantly, that the nurse is frequently more embarrassed by some procedure than the patient. Disparity in the nurse-patient relationship and its consequences should be given wider recognition in nurse training. It is often emphasised that nurses should try to understand their patient's embarrassment but there should be more of an attempt to understand the position of the nurse and the reasons for any unease she may be feeling. As I have suggested, the dependence of the patient (at least the male patient) may give rise to some resentment against the female nurse and the anomaly she represents—power held by the female. At the same time the patient may enjoy some aspects of his enforced dependence in a quasi-sexual way. Nurses can be well aware of these feelings but are currently offered little help in dealing with them.

Challenging nurse stereotypes

Recent contributors to nursing journals have complained that nurses are increasingly concerned with their image and not sufficiently interested in their principal role of caring for the patient. Some see any examination of nursing images as 'navel-gazing' or a sign of nursing becoming 'too political' (see Jones 1985). But nursing is, among other things, a political issue. All too often the stereotypes of nurses actually interfere with nurses doing their job. Moreover they may prevent us from realising opportunities to acquire a powerful voice in the promotion of health. In order to provide a high standard of care, nursing has first to put its own house in order. This includes addressing the issue of the public image of nurses, with all the potential effects this has on nursing morale, on the self-image of individual nurses, on the relationship between nursing and medicine and nurses and doctors and, finally, between nurses and patients.

The development of nursing is seriously hindered by many of the common images of nurses. The representation of the nurse as handmaiden or as sexual plaything undermines nursing as a responsible occupation. Nurses are not only portrayed as inevitably promiscuous but the implication is that they have no qualms about walking away from their responsibilities for a bit of slap and tickle in the linen cupboard. Or the image of the nurse as someone who searches among her patients or medical colleagues for a mate suggests nursing is just a side-line, a means to other ends.

In addition, the study of nursing stereotypes is important because misleading representations of nurses create expectations which cannot be met in real life. The term 'reality shock' has been used to describe the experience of the nursing recruit for whom the image of nurse-as-angel is suddenly seen as a lie, but it could equally be applied to the experience of the layperson-turned-patient. This is especially the case where shortages of staff and supplies are undermining the human qualities of nursing staff, let alone any superhuman ones. Recognising how images of nurses are constructed is also important in understanding the nurse-patient relationship and, for example, reactions to nursing procedures that in some way impinge on the sexuality of nurse or patient.

The extent to which *nurses* can have an impact on stereotyping is, of course, debatable; representations of nurses are constructed outside nursing as much as within. Some nurses (such as those who appeared in *Playboy* in the United States) have actually reinforced one public image of nurses. Others are taking direct action to challenge this kind of stereotyping by picketing cinemas showing pornographic films about nurses, for example, or by trying to get their unions to start campaigning about public images of the nurse. Certainly, the extent to which some images may be perpetuated *within* nursing can be mitigated by acknowledgement of their effects, so that stereotypes are dealt with collectively by nurses rather than struggled with at an individual level. Schools of nursing could do much to make nurses examine their own implicit stereotypes as well as to prepare them to deal with the effects of popular images on their work. This applies as much to clichés concerning the nurse-doctor relationship as to those of the nurse-patient relationship.

The specific image of the nurse as doctor's handmaiden is being challenged but at the same time there is a strange enthusiasm for extending the role of the nurse by taking over from doctors tasks which they themselves find mundane or tiresome (such as taking blood, or putting up intravenous infusions). Ironically, accepting these tasks brings nursing increasingly under the authority of doctors although they are taken on in a move to improve the status of nursing. Cheek by jowl with this has been an acceptance of medical input into nurse training with the sense that lectures given by doctors are somehow intrinsically better than those given by nurses.

What is needed is for the situation to be turned on its head, and ways created of introducing more nursing input into medical education. Only then might the doctor-nurse relationship radically change at a practical level. The concept of nurse as handmaiden persists partly because many doctors are unaware of what nursing is or could be and in what ways it is independent of medicine. Nurse tutors therefore must push for opportunities to offer formal lectures to medical students on current nursing philosophy, the historical relationship between nursing and medicine and the way in which nursing now perceives itself in relation to medicine. In addition there should be joint seminars for nursing and medical students to discuss their different contributions to patient care and to foster understanding of how nurses and doctors can best collaborate. Nurses also need to evaluate carefully any proposals to extend their clinical role and assess whether suggested duties fall within the province of nursing (as currently defined) or are essentially those of a medical aide.

7

Sexuality, the nurse and the patient

Introduction

One of the reasons why sexual health care is not incorporated into nursing is because of problems inherent in the nurse-patient relationship itself. The sexuality of the nurse or patient is often an integral part of the relationship, although this disquieting element is generally ignored. Widespread notions about women in general and popular images of male and female nurses play a role here, and in the first part of this chapter some of the consequences of these stereotypes emerge. In addition, the very nature of nursing—the physical and emotional intimacy it involves—makes certain demands not only on the patient (as discussed earlier) but also on nurses. This chapter will examine the use of expressive touch and the carrying out of intimate procedures as two of the ways in which the sexuality of the nurse and patient are implicated. Sexuality also becomes an issue if it is closely linked to the patient's status. This is more obvious where the patient's presenting condition (for example, unwanted pregnancy or sexually transmitted disease) has a clear association with sexuality. It is less obvious if the lifestyle or morality of the patient are different from, and in some way challenge, that of the nurse. Finally, sexuality becomes evident within the nurse-patient relationship where there is any genuine attempt to provide patient privacy. Not only does privacy potentially allow the patient to be sexually expressive, thereby raising several problems for the nurse, but the option of privacy in itself changes the terms of the nurse-patient relationship. All these instances can be seen as part of the general back-drop to the process of nursing and may subtly influence the every-day behaviour and reactions of the nurse.

Sexuality and the nurse-patient relationship

There are a number of ways in which the sexuality of the nurse or the patient may enter into the nurse-patient relationship. To begin with, as we have already seen, body-image, body-boundary and self-concept are significant aspects of sexuality in both health and illness. These phenomena are also, of course, important in nurses' personal lives and, to some extent, at work. We have seen how popular portrayals of nurses (for example in novels and on television) attribute certain qualities to individual nurses regard-less of their personal attributes or deficiencies. As a result, many nurses are acutely aware that once they appear publicly as nurses they become an object to be gazed at and projected on to. As one nurse I spoke to put it:

'Walking on to the ward was a strange thing. I felt very self-conscious—but it was a different feeling going on to a men's ward. As a woman I think you are anyway aware of being watched by men, of being evaluated by your appearance. The men's ward was like the world outside although in some ways more intense.'

But whether a ward is for men or women the visibility of the nurse, the sense of being 'on-stage' can in itself be difficult to deal with. One staff nurse told me:

'My first ward was the eye ward and I really enjoyed that. Looking back, it was easier *because* people couldn't see. They mostly had eye-pads on and I never experienced that embar-rassment I was to find on the next ward. I was really unpre-pared for the huge open space that one had to walk on to—a bit like walking on to a stage.'

Being so visible also seems to heighten the way nurses feel about potentially embarrassing aspects of their work, such as dealing with excreta, as this nurse recalls:

'A part of me always felt it was rather demeaning to be dealing with other people's waste products. I wouldn't mind carrying an empty bedpan, but to carry a full one was rather different. And to be seen by someone you half-fancied when you were doing the bottle round was an odd combination of roles and feelings.'

As this nurse suggests, the way in which nurses' sexuality has long been emphasised and exploited means that nursing tasks which may in themselves, be embarrassing to some degree for nurse and patient, become all the more so because of the sexual imagery attached to nurses.

There is generally some acknowledgement in nurse training of the initial embarrassment nurses may feel about some aspects of their work, but for the most part the emphasis is on the patient's discomfort. This fails to acknowledge that nurses in training are often less experienced in the ways of the world and may be more embarrassed by the intimate nature of their work than many of their patients. The majority of nurses I spoke to found that the embarrassment they experience when undertaking routine procedures diminishes with time, but never really resolves itself. Interestingly, it is not only confined to situations where men nurse women or women nurse men. However, the majority of nurses I spoke to found themselves most embarrassed when nursing patients of the opposite sex who were of their own age. This was regardless of the nurse's sexual preference or whether they experienced sexual attraction to a particular patient. More seemed to depend on the possible interpretation the *patient* might place on the relationship. This seems to suggest that the power relations existing between nurse and patient are more complex than is often realised; in some situations at least, the patient holds considerable power *vis-à-vis* the nurse. This is more clearly the case where the patient has realised the vulnerability of the nurse and insists on making sexuality an issue, if only jokingly.

Embarrassment is a reasonable reaction to a breach of the usual social conventions but it also reflects the power relations between nurse and patient. The nurses I spoke to realised that although they often felt embarrassed about aspects of their work, this was easier to deal with when caring for those patients most heavily dependent on nursing care—in other words where the roles of nurse and patient are clearest cut, and the nurse's power undisputed. Similarly, in situations where there is little ambiguity of role, nurses are often sufficiently uninhibited to trade overtly on the stereotype and use their sexuality to oil the wheels of the nurse-patient relationship. They may, for example, encourage compliance with nursing procedures by coquettishly pleading with the patient to be co-operative 'just for me', by the use of innuendo and the pretence of sexual attraction.

Sexual attraction

Genuine sexual attraction is an obvious way in which sexuality may enter into the nurse-patient relationship, with attraction experienced either by one or both parties. Such feelings are inevitable from time to time, although for a nurse to admit as much is still considered a terrible breach of professional behaviour. To sweep this issue under the carpet, however, is counterproductive. Clearly, different people will deal with sexual attraction in different ways but the confusion that may be experienced by the nurse who is attracted to her patient can interfere with the provision of good nursing care. The nurse may, for example, make a poor nursing assessment because the same questions which seem to have relevance in the assessment of other patients now seem unduly personal and difficult to ask. Carrying out nursing procedures can also become difficult where there is personal attraction. Just taking a patient's pulse, for instance, can become a highly charged action. Nurses often deal with the 'problem' of sexual attraction by avoiding the patient as much as possible or by adopting an offhand manner. Some nurses will react in almost the opposite fashion, becoming closely involved with their patient and reluctant to allow him or her space to regain their independence.

Sexual attraction is a fact of life, and will inevitably become an issue for most nurses at some time or other, but there is no way of stipulating how it should be dealt with. Much will depend on the individual personalities involved and on the overall context, such as the degree of patient dependence. But judging from the response of nurses I spoke to, what would be helpful—at least for some nurses—would be somewhere to go for support in dealing with this issue. As one student said:

'When I worked on the children's ward I was looking after a lad of seventeen. He just sat in his room all day getting bored. I found him really attractive and as soon as I went into the room and started talking to him, I just couldn't look at him. I was like

a little schoolgirl really! And I found that really difficult—
trying to talk to him and nurse him—and I wished there was
someone I could have talked to about it.'

Seduction

Attraction is not only experienced by nurses. Patients may also be
attracted to those who nurse them and, depending on how this is
expressed, their behaviour may affect the kind of care they
receive. However, as Whitley (1978) points out, not all patient behaviour signalling attraction necessarily means what it suggests; it
may represent nothing more than an attempt to validate sexual
identity where this has been undermined by ill health. For many
people, recovering from illness involves finding confirmation of
their attractiveness as a sexual being and they may seek this from
nurses. This apparently seductive behaviour is quite different
from an invitation to a sexual relationship of some sort.

According to Whitley, nurses should treat seductive behaviour
not as a social invitation but as a nursing issue. In practical terms
this means the nurse should 'qualify' such behaviour (by, for
example, the careful use of voice tone, avoidance of unnecessary
touch or little eye contact). By these means she demonstrates
neither disapproval nor encouragement, but neutrality. At the
same time, she should recognise the needs that underlie the
patient's behaviour and 'redirect' him by encouraging him to express his real concerns. While Whitley makes an important point,
it should also be recognised that there can be a fine line between
seductive behaviour and sexual harassment.

Sexual harassment

Sexual harassment seems to be something of an occupational
hazard, particularly for female nurses. Sexual harassment at work
has been defined as unwarranted verbal or sexual advances which
interfere with the employee's work, job security or prospects. It
can also refer to a work environment laden with sex-stereotyped
attitudes and behaviour which emphasise the employee's sexuality and degrade her role as a worker (Hadjifotiou 1983). Female
nurses may experience both forms of harassment. Many are
'jokingly' asked to climb into their patients' beds. Others have

known patients to use touch in an ambiguous but, for the most part, suggestive way. Some nurses have had to cope with the patient's deliberate exposure of his erect penis (as opposed to the unintentional erection that may occur during a nursing procedure), or even with sexual assault. Nurses may also experience sexual harassment from male colleagues—especially, it seems, from doctors who think they can ignore the female nurse as colleague and exploit her instead as a woman and handmaiden.

There is unfortunately a long tradition in which male doctors emphasise female nurses' sexuality and, in doing so, degrade their specific contribution to health care. Sadly, this tradition is very slow to change. Only recently, for example, a general practitioner wrote in the medical press suggesting how to treat hypothermia. This GP had heard of a patient with a core temperature of only 26° C whose condition had failed to improve using conventional measures (Norwell 1986). A geriatrician therefore put into effect 'the King David regime'; the patient's normal temperature was restored by a 'nineteen-year-old, warm-blooded nurse' who 'in true Nightingale style' slipped into bed with the patient. The author concludes with the suggestion that male patients at this hospital have been asking their visitors for ice and low reading thermometers instead of grapes. Apart from the dismal predictability of this final comment, what is significant is the seemingly unquestioned authority of a doctor to ask a nurse to perform what is, after all, a very personal service, and to classify this as a part of nursing tradition. It has to be said that *if* such physical contact offered the only chance of recovery for the patient, it did not necessarily have to be supplied by a young, female nurse. There is nothing to stop doctors offering this sort of service themselves—assuming of course that they are warm-blooded!

It seems that doctors will continue to treat nurses as handmaidens and sex objects until effectively challenged by nurses. This means that nurse tutors have a particular responsibility for the way they directly or indirectly describe the nurse-doctor relationship to their students. It also means that nurses, both qualified and unqualified, must become more assertive in their dealings with doctors whenever the role and dignity of the individual nurse are undermined (see final chapter). It further means that nurses must be prepared to become involved in medical training and to take every opportunity to clarify for medical students what nursing does and does not involve.

Intimate procedures

The so-called 'King David regime' involved some sexual innuendo for Norwell. However, more orthodox nursing procedures can carry a different, but nonetheless sexual, charge for either the nurse or patient involved. Take, for example, the task of giving a patient a suppository. This involves a violation of the patient's body-image and the integrity of his body-boundary as well as an assault on his sense of privacy and dignity. In addition, the nurse gains a specific 'knowledge' of the patient that would probably be withheld from most other people—if not *everyone* else. The nurse is at some level aware of intruding into the patient's privacy, of physical entry into the body, perhaps the self, of the patient. The nurse is also aware of his or her technical ability (or lack of it) and the patient's expectation that a nurse will handle the situation with assurance. As we saw in Chapter 1, whether or not an action is interpreted as sexual depends on the context and the intention of the actor. It is therefore for the nurse—essentially through proficiency—to clarify the reality of the situation, to show that the intention is to carry out a nursing procedure and not a sexual act.

Emerson (1971) has studied this sort of tacit understanding as it exists in the doctor-patient relationship, and her work can be usefully extended to cover the interaction between nurse and patient. Emerson looked at the behaviour expected of patients and doctors during gynaecological examinations and how this behaviour has to demonstrate that the examination is a clinical investigation and not a sexual violation. Doctors, she found, are obliged by some sort of unspoken understanding to be seen to divorce the part of the body under examination from the person inhabiting the body. They transform the body into a technical object to be worked on and ignore the total person that it represents.

One way of doing this is to look past the patient while the vaginal examination takes place, avoiding all eye contact. The patient is expected to comply by avoiding the eye of the gynaecologist, and refraining from conversation which might reintroduce a sense of herself as a person. She is expected to behave with great decorum both before and after the examination; to do otherwise would suggest lewdness. However, she must throw modesty to the winds *during* the procedure itself and expose her genitals to one or more strangers without protest. To do otherwise would draw attention to herself and, again, reintroduce her personality. Only with these safeguards, Emerson claims, can the examination be experienced by both parties as unambiguously part of a world of professional concern and personal disinterest.

All intimate procedures present the difficulty of treating patients with consideration while demonstrating the non-sexual nature of nurses' actions. Strategies such as those described by Emerson, lack of eye contact, for example, are widely, if unconsciously, applied and can be helpful in confirming the non-sexual nature of the procedure, but they can also create an impression of offhandedness or lack of concern. This aspect of nursing procedure should be given wider recognition in nurse training. Nurses need to discuss whether such strategies are really necessary, or whether the non-sexual nature of intimate procedures can be clearly defined by other, less depersonalising measures.

Significantly, the strategies described by Emerson have evolved because ambiguity is otherwise experienced not just by the patient but also by the health worker. So in the same way that a patient may need reassurance, the nurse may also need to know that his or her actions will not be misinterpreted in sexual terms. Moreover, nurses are vulnerable in that the very way in which they undertake an intimate procedure can reveal a great deal about them, not just as nurses but also as people and sexual beings. It is as if there is some sort of connection between the nurse's sexuality and his or her confidence and proficiency as a nurse, as the following quote demonstrates:

'Having had smears done myself, I know it makes you feel very vulnerable and exposed. Your anatomy is available for criticism and comparison. So is your response to being examined. When it comes to *doing* smears, your concerns are different but there's still that vulnerability. You wonder "Am I making them feel uncomfortable? Do they feel I'm technically clumsy? How do I appear to be responding to their anatomy? Do they feel dissatisfied because I haven't done it well in their terms?" It's a very odd thing and never really talked about but it's not just your ability that's being challenged but—in both instances really—[having a smear done and taking a smear] your sexuality is somehow on the line.' (Family planning nurse)

This suggests that the sexuality of both nurse and patient are threatened by the procedure, albeit in different ways. Again, nurses need to be able to discuss the problems raised by intimate procedures and to develop strategies which are helpful for both patients and nurses.

Touch and the cost of caring

It has been well recognised that the nursing process encourages greater intimacy between nurses and patients (see, for example, Salvage 1985). Because the patient is seen as an individual rather than an illness, and because nurses do not flit from patient to patient as they tended to do with task allocation, they have become less well-defended and more emotionally involved. To accept the nurse's vulnerability as well as the patient's, to acknowledge that the distinction between their two worlds is not necessarily clear-cut, means we must reconsider how we should understand nursing itself as a process and what is meant by some of the fundamentals, such as the concept of care.

As Kitson (1985) has pointed out, much of nursing care depends on reaching out and supporting people who are anxious or frightened. While this aspect of nursing care has been delineated from even vaguer notions of 'care' as the concept of 'nurse-patient communication', little attention has been given to the way in which this kind of communication can be integrated into nursing as a whole. Kitson suggests this is perhaps because there is no space within either the nursing curriculum or ward protocol for recognising the way in which nurses have to become, to some extent, emotionally involved with their patients *in order* to care. It is certainly expected of nurses that they will meet the emotional needs of their patients (what Kitson calls 'the hidden curriculum'), but the realities of how they should actually do this in practice are ignored.

The extent of nurses' involvement has recently become a contentious issue. In the past nurses were discouraged from entering their patient's world. In fact, the nurse's separateness from the patient was regarded as a sign of professionalism. Very slowly, however, things have changed. The dinstinction between the worlds of the patient and the nurse has become blurred and yet little attention has been given to the meaning or effects of such a lack of distinction (Gow 1982). This is clearly demonstrated, for example, by the way in which nurses are being encouraged to use touch. In Chapter 2 I briefly discussed the importance of touch from a patient's perspective. Here I want to look at it more from the nurse's position as influenced by the nurse-patient relationship.

Touch between nurses and patients has been classified into two different kinds. First there is 'instrumental touch' which is an inevitable part of nursing, for example in lifting a patient or taking a pulse. Touch in this form is supposedly impersonal but nonetheless contributes to the ambiguity which may be sensed in intimate procedures. We are more concerned here with the second type—'expressive touch'. This is a spontaneous form of touch arising from an emotional response to a patient's situation and open to influence by a number of factors.

While touch undoubtedly has the potential to be the most meaningful form of communication between nurses and patients, its use involves considerable risk. Barnett (1972b) has found touch can be misinterpreted up to half the time by either nurse or patient. As a result, the spontaneous use of touch may be inhibited in situations where the risk of misinterpretation is greatest, for example where patients are nursed in private rooms or private households. The age, sex, culture and class status of the individuals concerned may also affect their attitude towards touch. Barnett (1972a) finds that 'affluent' patients are touched less than others—unsurprising given that the ability of freedom to touch is generally associated with the degree of power an individual holds (Henley 1973). This can be seen from the way that a male consultant surgeon or physician appears to feel fairly free to touch his female nurse colleagues while nurses are not in an equally free position to respond or actually initiate touch themselves. (How many times have you seen a student nurse put her arm around a consultant?) Correspondingly, nurses' use of touch in relation to their patients has to be seen, at least to some extent, in terms of the degree of power they hold *vis-à-vis* a particular patient. On this basis, a wealthy patient—or a sick nurse tutor—may be difficult to touch.

While nurses may be inhibited by some contexts, it also remains fairly easy to patronise patients by the indiscriminate use of touch. Therefore it is important for nurses to examine their motivation for touching or wanting to touch their patients; it may not be purely sympathy they wish to convey (Ujhely 1979). Moreover, there are times when touch may be unwelcome if not actually distressing and the thoughtless use of touch on the part of the nurse may suppress the patient's own expression of emotion. Hall (1966) notes how in times of disaster, the need to avoid physical contact can be crucial for some people. As someone recently bereaved told me:

> 'I felt as if my very core—what *should* have been deep inside of me—was now on the outside. And the outside that could usually safely respond to touch was now inside. Because I felt turned inside-out I couldn't bear for anyone to touch me. The most innocent touch became so strongly charged it was frightening.'

It is clear that there are no standard ways in which expressive touch can be employed; it is a spontaneous action arising from very specific circumstances and cannot be governed by a fixed set of rules. Instead the use of expressive touch by the nurse represents a balance between a nurse's emotional response to a particular patient's circumstances and judgement of what is an appropriate form of communication in a specific situation.

Unfortunately, however, there are moves within nursing to attempt some sort of standardisation in the use of expressive touch. Paradoxically, this arises in part from the recognition of the positive uses of touch. Touch is increasingly seen as an aid to healing, and its use opens up exciting possibilities for the development of nursing (see for example Krieger 1975). Of course, the use of touch as encouraged by humanistic nurses is not of a standardised form. Many nurses who attempt to use touch therapeutically work intuitively rather than from a set of rules. There are, however, those who tend to take some of the principles underlying this approach out of context and attempt to make them more formal.

Goodykoontz (1979), writing about geriatric nursing, argues that if technology has little to offer the elderly, nurses—through touch—can offer *themselves* as well as their hands. According to Goodykoontz, the spontaneous use of touch can diminish the distance between nurse and patient and there is no incompatibility between appearing both warm and concerned and competent. She also argues, less convincingly, perhaps, that even if the nurse is not a person who generally uses touch, she should try to overcome this tendency when putting on the 'cloak of a nurse' for fear the patient might otherwise feel rejected. Ujhely (*ibid*) also suggests we should reach out to a patient as the situation demands— even if the nurse is not genuinely moved by a patient's distress. Susannah Wright sees nurses as fulfilling the role of a mother for their patients and part of this role, she feels, ought to be the hold-ing, hugging and physical reassurance of the patient. A mother 'communicates with her body the warmth and security the child needs'—except in this instance it is the patient-as-child who needs security (1985).

There are problems in the views mentioned above, at least from the nurse's perspective. First of all, it does not seem a good idea for nurses to model their role on that of the mother. It brings us right back to the image of nursing as women's work and women as nurturers. Do we, for example, look to male nurses to give warmth and security to their patients *through their bodies* or is it that we expect women (as opposed to nurses *per se*) to provide this sort of comfort? Second, although this is not an entirely separate point, nurses are only human and can only give so much. There is a place within nursing for expressive touch but it cannot become a tenet of nursing that the nurse *should* touch or hold patients according to some preformulated plan. Expressive touch arises from empathy and from a genuine regard for the person one is moved to touch.

> 'I know you can feel—either when you give or receive touch—whether it's authentic and that's what's important. It matters that you are moving from a place of caring. People feel only more isolated if you touch them because you're supposed to do it.'   (Nurse/Massage therapist)

Unfortunately it is not possible for nurses to *like* all their patients, and without some basic liking it is rare for expressive touch to manifest itself. Once touch is not spontaneous, it cannot be expres-sive, only an empty gesture. It cannot be demanded that all nurses should in principle be prepared to hold all their patients. Inevit-ably, individual nurses will only feel able to give expressive touch to a small number of patients—to suggest otherwise is almost to suggest that nursing is a form of prostitution. It is also subtly to endorse the madonna/whore role attributed to women in general and to female nurses in particular.

I am not advocating that the nurse should stand aloof when a patient is distressed—hopefully all of us are genuinely moved at some level by the distress of others. But there is all the difference in the world between providing a reassuring touch *or* word and being asked automatically to embrace a patient, actually to take someone in your arms, even when you feel uneasy about 'giving' yourself in this way.

Touch can be a positive, healing force or it can be damaging or distressing. Much depends on who is doing the touching, who is being touched, the type of touch used and the overall context. Unfortunately, as we have seen, some nurses writing about touch ignore the importance of context and intuition. The sort of guidelines Ujhely and Goodykoontz suggest, for example (referred to earlier), are similar in tone to the question frequently voiced at nursing conferences and in the nursing press, 'Nurse, do you care enough?'. In the case of touch, the underlying assumption is that if you care enough you will be prepared to give of yourself both physically and emotionally to all your patients. Not only does this suggest that care can be a simple matter of fingering the patient, but there is also the danger that the nurse will be 'guilt-tripped' into standardised but questionable behaviour, instead of being allowed to form and act on her own judgement. This judgement is not an innate quality but comes largely from experience, and needs to be nurtured by proper training and the good example of more experienced staff.

The use of expressive touch can present problems for nurses as well as patients. It is not always appropriate and, even where it is, its costs can be heavy. The use of touch can elicit strong emotion. It is therefore important that nurses who use this form of touch and give much of themselves by doing so should also be given support.

The blurring of any strong distinction between the patient's and the nurse's worlds might be an important factor in the development of a new identity for nursing—in, for example, the trend towards nursing as patient advocacy. However, it is not without difficulties for the nurse. Moreoever the support required by any move of this sort involves more than is obvious at first glance. Nurses cannot be asked to *care*—with everything this is coming to imply—unless they can take support not only from their peers but also from more senior staff who, in effect, are demanding of them that they care enough. Before this level of support will be sought or forthcoming though, the attitudes of senior nurses and indeed the very hierarchical nature of nursing will have to be changed. No-one, for example, will seek help from a more senior nurse when this might be thought to indicate an inability to cope and therefore come to prejudice further employment. Nor will nurses seek support from those they feel have become unfamiliar with and unsympathetic towards the practical day-to-day problems associated with their job. In other words, if nurses are to deal with the 'hidden curriculum' and begin to meet the emotional needs of their patients, nurse managers and tutors will have to become less grade-conscious and more accessible and supportive.

Nurses and homosexuality

Another way in which the boundary between the worlds of nurse and patient becomes blurred is where the patient's circumstances or way of life pose a direct threat or challenge to aspects of the nurse's sexuality, for example when a patient is known or thought to be homosexual. The attitudes of many nurses towards homosexuality are probably similar to those of a large section of the general population and generally expressed as *homophobia* (fear or hatred of those attracted to the same sex). One nurse told me his peers saw homosexuality as 'yet another mark of this society going to hell'. Most nurses either censure or ignore homosexuality and it seems that nurse education is doing little to change this. With regard to nurse training I was told:

'Homosexuality was brushed over. It was discussed that you go through that stage when you're a teenager and you have a crush on somebody and that some people remain homosexual, but it wasn't discussed any deeper than that. It was sort of assumed that everyone in the room wasn't homosexual.'

For one reason or another, nursing patients who are known or thought to be homosexual raises problems for some nurses. This may be because the nurse is also homosexual and fears victimisation if it becomes known. He or she may be reminded of this by the attitudes of other nurses to homosexual patients. Alternatively, in the light of what was said earlier—that few people are exclusively homosexual or heterosexual—the majority of people at times experience attraction to people of the same sex, but are aware of the climate which dictates we must have either one sexual preference or another (and preferably not the other!). It is therefore extremely confusing for the person who sees themself as exclusively heterosexual to experience a shift from social and personal norms.

They may well prefer to ignore this confusion but contact with anyone known to be homosexual may make this difficult. There is also the view that homosexuality is inherently 'bad' and in a sense contagious; homosexuality is imagined by some to 'spread' through the 'corruption' of the young or others who are supposedly vulnerable to the sexual advances of homosexuals. Yet there is no reason to believe that a person will choose a different sexuality because of the example of another person (Beer *et al.* 1983).

Nurses' attitudes towards gay patients have been described by Pongoncheff (1979). She found, for example, that a lesbian patient was given poor nursing care because the nursing staff felt so uneasy about her sexuality (and presumably their own too). This patient, who was admitted with thrombophlebitis, was given little attention other than her prescribed medications. Her calls for assistance often went unanswered, back rubs or help with turning were given only grudgingly and visits by her lover prompted giggling among the staff and the exchange of 'knowing glances'. Furthermore, her lover was treated with coldness by staff and denied the usual general information given to friends or relatives about a patient's progress. The atmosphere was such that the patient discharged herself and this finally prompted the staff to examine their attitudes. With hindsight they acknowledged that they had gossiped about the patient and discussed confidential information in a way that had compromised the patient's privacy and prejudiced members of the staff against her. They had to admit that their 'mood of conspiracy' had also affected the attitudes of other patients. In addition, the staff had denied the patient basic nursing care.

Looking at *why* they had behaved in such a way, it emerged that individual nurses had felt awkward about touching the patient in an intimate way. They felt uneasy about being alone with her behind drawn curtains. One of the principal reasons for this turned out to be fear that the patient might make some sexual advance to them and they would not know how to respond. Once they had recognised this fear they realised how ridiculous it was: a lesbian patient is no more likely to make a 'pass' than any other patient and indeed is probably less likely to do so because of her vulnerable position. Nurses also felt threatened by a lifestyle so different from their own, saying it made them think about issues they just did not want to face. There was also particular fear among female nurses that if they appeared to accept lesbianism, their own sexuality would be placed in question.

Pongoncheff felt that the discussion of attitudes among these nurses would probably mean they would deal with similar situations more successfully in the future. For example, the nurses came up with the following suggestions:

1. that it should not be assumed that the patient is as confused about sexuality as the nurse;
2. that homosexual patients and their visiting lovers should be given sufficient privacy, but in a way that does not draw attention to them or make their fellow patients uncomfortable;
3. that most problems which arise within the nursing of homosexual patients probably stem from the attitudes of the staff. While attitudes cannot be changed overnight, staff can still provide good nursing care while attempting to come to terms with their attitudes.

The first step in changing attitudes, according to Pongoncheff, is through self-awareness. The nurse should take time to discover what her attitudes are, and if she is disturbed by the concept of homosexuality, she should try to define what she finds so threatening. The nurse should also examine what she knows about homosexuality and what she is merely assuming. Nurses should remember that their attitudes can be indicated to the patient before they themselves are aware of their patient's sexuality, simply, for example, by the way in which they phrase questions in taking a history. As Pongoncheff has said, it cannot be assumed that all patients are 'straight' any more than it can be assumed that all married patients have monogamous relationships. By avoiding such terms as 'wife' or 'husband', for example, and substituting 'partner', or by the use of pronouns which do not imply an assumption of the sex of the partner, the nurse allows patients space to be open about their sexuality if they so wish. These guidelines may be especially helpful for the nurse working with people who have AIDS.

AIDS and sexuality

Acquired Immune Deficiency Syndrome (AIDS) draws attention to sexual lifestyle perhaps more than any other disease that may be sexually transmitted. A number of issues may be raised for those nursing people with AIDS.

Contrary to some beliefs, the disease is not restricted to people of a particular sexual persuasion. However in Britain the largest proportion of all cases of AIDS—about 90 per cent—is presently reported among male homosexuals or bisexuals. Consequently although not everyone who contracts AIDS is gay, AIDS has become synonymous with homosexuality. In addition to this, partly because homosexuals are stereotyped as promiscuous and partly because educational campaigns stress that the risk of getting AIDS increases with the number of sexual partners a person has, AIDS has additionally become identified with promiscuity. This is despite the fact that the disease can be transmitted by non-sexual means (such as blood transfusion), by only one sexual encounter with an infected person or by sex with a supposedly monogamous partner. Because of the popular image of AIDS which ignores these facts, a diagnosis of AIDS is often interpreted as an indisputable statement about sexual behaviour. This statement moreover concerns modes of behaviour outside many nurses' experience and which therefore promote unease. It is not the only reason though why nursing people with AIDS poses particular problems.

The nature of the disease and the absence of any cure makes fear of AIDS understandable. Yet fear has also been needlessly elaborated and extended to include people as well as the disease. It has, for example, escalated into a paranoia which sees all gay men as potential carriers of the AIDS virus. Consequently homophobia has increased to a point where some groups (for instance, the so-called Moral Majority in America) are advocating the isolation of all homosexuals as a way of controlling AIDS (see Patton 1985). For others, the initial identification of AIDS with homosexuality in the West is seen as divine retribution for a form of behaviour they consider a perversion. An analogy has been drawn, for instance, between AIDS and the Plague which, in its time, was also interpreted as just punishment for an evil world. One of the problems with this way of thinking is that it understands homosexuality rather than any virus to be the cause of AIDS. It also ignores the fact that a large group of homosexuals, namely lesbians, are thought to be less at risk of acquiring AIDS than many heterosexuals. What is happening is that 'AIDS is being used by a heterosexist society as an excuse to moralise on the lives of those who disagree with its basic premise' (McAllister 1985).

At another level, fear of acquiring AIDS from a *known* carrier of the virus appears to be heightened where the person is homosexual—as if the gay person with AIDS is highly contagious. Aids is not a contagious disease in the sense of being transmitted by touch although it is widely understood to be so. Homosexuality, we saw earlier, is also thought to be contagious in some strange way. The homosexual person with AIDS therefore becomes a doubly dangerous character for the uninformed.

Nurses are often as guilty of this particular form of prejudice as anyone else, but their attitudes towards people with AIDS may also be heavily influenced by fears of acquiring the disease because of the nature of their work. AIDS *is* frightening because it is transmissible but, contrary to the fears of many health workers, the risk to those working with people with AIDS or those with antibodies to the AIDS virus comes not from mere contact with such patients but from carelessness in the handling of waste products and from accidental self-inoculation from used 'sharps'. According to the DHSS, although the virus responsible for AIDS (Human Immunodeficiency Virus or HIV) has been found in blood, semen, tears, breast milk and saliva, infection appears to principally transmitted by sexual intercourse or by the transfusion or inoculation of contaminated blood or blood products. A DHSS report makes it clear that there is no evidence that social contact with antibody-positive individuals—such as the sharing of eating utensils or toilet facilities—presents a risk of infection (1986). So far, no health care worker in the world is known to have acquired AIDS from a patient, although there are instances where staff have developed HIV antibodies following a sharps injury (*British Medical Journal* 1986). It is understandable that nurses should wish to protect themselves against AIDS as far as possible but there are dangers in overdoing this. For example, according to the DHSS (*ibid*), health personnel need to wear gloves, masks, plastic aprons, overgowns and eye protection only if there is a risk of contamination with the AIDS virus during invasive anaesthetic, surgical or dental procedures. For simple clinical procedures, including the handling of blood or other body fluids, only gloves and plastic aprons need be worn. And yet nurses have been known to dress in full protective regalia, including overshoes, simply to deliver a cup of tea to a patient with AIDS! Imagine how this must undermine the patient's self-concept, especially at a time when the patient's whole world, including other aspects of sexuality, are already under serious threat. Moreover, overdressing of this sort may be counterproductive in that the nurse comes to depend on protective clothing rather than safe practice. It is in just this sort of situation that accidental self-inoculation with the AIDS virus may occur through, for example, careless handling of used needles. According to the RCN AIDS Working Party Report (1986b) AIDS, more than any other disease in recent years, has underlined the inability of many nurses to meet their patients' emotional needs. This deficiency is seen to result from a fundamental failure in basic nurse education which is inadequate in the way it attempts to promote counselling skills, encourage development of interpersonal relationships, or provide the basis for understanding different lifestyles. The attitudes of nursing staff can have a dramatic influence on the psychological state of the person with AIDS. They may, for example, influence the readiness or ability of nurses to allow patients to discuss aspects of lifestyle or to give specific information which may enhance or help to protect, such as the principles of safer sex.

A homosexual man with AIDS suffers problems over and above those directly caused by the disease. He may have been keeeping his sexual identity secret, but his right to privacy about his sexual preference may be seriously undermined by the diagnosis of AIDS. This in turn may put his job or his relationships with family or friends at risk. Such patients are in need of a great deal of support as well as information from nursing staff. The RCN Working Party on AIDS has raised the point (applicable to any long-term relationship outside marriage) of the necessity of nurses to accept the right of patients to define their own next of kin, despite the difficulties this may pose for nurses and for the patient's family. According to the Chairman of the working party, Richard Wells, 'it was our way of saying that the patient should retain control, not only of his own life but in helping the partner to maintain control as well'.

While there is a move within nursing to recognise the role of grieving in bereavement, this recognition is often not extended to the lover of the person with AIDS; the lack of support partners receive from friends and health workers on the death of their lover can affect their future relationships, their future sexuality and possibly the rest of their lives. Recognition of the lover as next of kin might bring increased recognition of his needs in bereavement. He may also be in need of support because of fears that he too has contracted AIDS. If nurses do not challenge their own prejudices and question their attitudes towards AIDS patients and their next of kin they will be failing to provide adequate nursing care.

Clearly nurses need an up-to-date understanding of AIDS and its mode of transmission as well as, in many cases, a change in attitude if they are to care for people with AIDS, whatever their sexual orientation. This will only come about with sound, broad-based training and regular up-dates to provide nurses not only with relevant information but also the opportunity to air their fears and examine their work practices in relation to their prejudices. (See also 'Further reading' at the end of this Chapter.)

Privacy

The provision of privacy represents a final example of how sexuality can influence the nurse-patient relationship. Privacy is important for patients for a number of reasons. It may, for example, be necessary for the patient to experience being alone. Privacy also allows conversations with visitors or staff that the patient does not wish others on the ward to hear. More controversially it is important if the patient is to be in any way sexually expressive.

Institutional life inevitably imposes some constraints on the provision of privacy. However, it seems there is remarkably little effort on the part of health workers to find the best possible solution to the problem of privacy within these limits. In fact it appears in the nurse's interests *not* to press for increased patient privacy.

Partial privacy can be provided by simply pulling curtains around a patient's bed, allowing even the illest patient the opportunity of physical closeness, often inhibited by an open ward. Curtains may also allow a silence between patient and visitor which might feel companionable in private but awkward in public. Curtains also, to some extent, muffle conversation. Yet despite the advantages offered by this simple measure, there is little acknowledgement of the right of the patient to claim his or her privacy in this way. One reason for this might be because it changes the dynamic of the nurse-patient relationship, and this may be difficult for the nurse to cope with. The nurse cannot assume open access to the patient, but must hesitate and think before disturbing a patient who has sought seclusion. Things are no longer solely on the nurse's terms. Remembering what has been said already about embarrassment indicating the locus of power in nurse-patient relationships, the words of one of the nurses I interviewed sum up the problem well. He spoke of a young patient who would draw the curtains when a visitor came: 'It was jolly embarrassing for all [nursing staff] because you'd be knocking on the curtain saying "Excuse me! Do you want your dinner now?" *It gets in the way!'*

Another and more effective source of privacy would be the provision of private rooms for patients to go to on their own or with visitors. These rooms could also provide the opportunity for sexual intimacy if desired. Some nurses, though, are even more uneasy about this suggestion than the proposal for the use of screens, and it is important to consider why. At the moment most hospitals are set up without a thought for patient privacy. To provide special rooms for patients would involve a change in priorities and planning. However, it is not these implications that worry the individual nurse. Nurses are to some extent accustomed to acting as custodians for their patients. They supervise their daily activities and treatments, often enforce a limitation on the number of visitors each will receive and, usually indirectly, they regulate the behaviour of patients and visitors. They carry out surveillance of their patients at a number of levels, monitoring not only temperature, pulse, respirations etc., but also the activities of the whole organism—including making sure that it is in the right place at the right time. Clearly, increased autonomy of the patient and the freedom to move out of range of the nurse's observation have implications for the custodial role of the nurse. Over and above this custodianship of the physical body is the sense that the nurse is the keeper of the patient's morality. And the idea of the patient wandering off for a bit of hanky-panky flies in the face of this unacknowledged aspect of the nurse's role.

The patient's morality is, of course, none of the nurse's business but an examination of the different values which exist in the private sector helps to demonstrate the flimsiness of any claim of nursing to moral guardianship. The private patient pays for privacy. There is no doubt that nurse-patient interaction is different in the private sector because of the obvious financial element in the relationship and it is difficult to see the nurse exerting the same custodial and inhibiting influence on sexual expression as she does in the NHS. At least the potential for sexual expression exists. Does this mean that sexual expression is morally wrong in the private sector but that the nurse as custodian has been 'bought off', or does it mean that the private patient's power of self-determination is greater simply because he or she is more obviously contributing financially towards his or her health care? In which case is it right that patients, because of their NHS status, are deprived of such self-determination?

> 'There should be private rooms, there should be quiet rooms where people can go and be together. Good God, we allow it in prison occasionally if it's warranted; why can't we allow it in the health care system?'   (Richard Wells, RCN)

Not all patients are going to be concerned about expressing the sexual aspect of their sexuality while an in-patient. But for those who are, it raises problems which involve not only the feelings of the patient and their visitor but also of fellow patients and staff. This issue is already being faced by some nurses. In some oncology units, for example, there is recognition of the sexual needs of patients. It is as if the nature of patients' diagnoses has thrown the important issues of life into focus and, as a result, patients, visitors and staff seem to respond to situations with more openness and flexibility.

One nurse, working in a paediatric oncology unit, spoke to me about the need to look at different developmental needs for different age groups. Peer-group support, for example, is extremely important in terms of a teenager's sexual development and therefore friends are actively encouraged to visit—if necessary in large gangs. At the same time, the nursing approach is family-centred, with parents as involved in the care of their child as they wish to be. Within this context, boyfriends or girlfriends of teenage patients are encouraged to visit and become involved in patient care or, where it is not in conflict with parents, in continuing or developing any sexual aspect of their relationship.

> 'We had one teenager who asked several of the nurses if his girl-friend could stay the night and he was actually in a single room ... I asked if he'd check it out with his parents or would he like

me to do it. He actually checked it out with them and they 'phoned back to say they'd no objection and she actually stayed the night. Obviously we talked to the night staff and they were quite happy about it.'

But in fact this was really only possible because of the level of discussion which regularly took place between staff and relatives and among staff members themselves in this unit. Things are very different on general wards where patients are admitted for a variety of reasons—some with life-threatening conditions, some with ingrowing toenails, some long-term patients, others just in for the day. Moreover real attention to the patient's need to express sexuality will not be possible where communication or mutual support among staff is poor.

This chapter has shown some of the ways in which sexuality forms an integral part of the nurse-patient relationship and indirectly helps to determine standards of care. The presence of sexuality is not always a problem but where it is there are no easy solutions. Problems are experienced at a personal, private level and all too often it is the individual nurse who is urged to take responsibility for change. It is she who should 'come to terms' with her sexuality, clarify her values, 'qualify' the behaviour of the patient. Yet many problems are beyond the scope of the individual nurse and need to be addressed by nursing as a whole. Nurses have become more emotionally involved with their patients, not only through personal choice but also as a result of the introduction of the nursing process and a shift of emphasis in nursing ideology. (The next chapter looks at sexuality in relation to nursing's theoretical stance in more detail.) To cope with this closer involvement and with the issues this chapter has raised, nurses need far more support than they currently receive. Just how this support can be given is discussed in the final chapter.

Further reading

RCN (1986b) *Nursing Guidelines on the Management of Patients in Hospital and the Community Suffering from AIDS: Second Report of the RCN AIDS Working Party.*

8

Avoiding theoretical confusion

We have seen how gender and sexuality create certain images and expectations of nurses which may indirectly affect standards of care. In this chapter we shall discuss the role of nursing theory (for example, concepts inherent in nurse education and research) in determining the kind of sexual health care nurses provide. There are at least two major problems in this area which have implications for the way nurses approach sexual health. One problem concerns the way in which sexuality itself is conceptualised; the basic understanding of sexuality which nurses try to apply is inadequate. The second problem concerns the use of nursing models. More precisely, there is confusion over how to apply models, leading to a limited assessment of patients' needs. Both problems restrict the kinds of goals nurses identify concerning the patient's sexual health. However, before looking at these issues in more detail it is important to place them in the context of a wider understanding of modern nursing theory.

Nursing theory

Nursing theory has blossomed in recent years. This is because, at one level, there is widespread recognition that nurses need a sound theoretical basis from which to develop nursing practice and plan nursing care. Underlying this, however, has been a strong desire to identify the essential elements of a nurse's practice that can be specifically recognised as nursing (as opposed to, for example, quasi-medical tasks). This suggests that the direction in which nursing theory is developing is partly shaped by the *political* goal of establishing an autonomy for nursing.

One way in which nursing attempts to differentiate itself from medicine is by claiming to be concerned with the patient who is ill rather than with the illness itself. Nursing claims to have a 'person orientation' which contrasts with the 'disease orientation' of orthodox medicine—a distinction, incidentally, which is denied by many medical practitioners. But whether or not nursing is more holistic in its approach than medicine, paradoxically, it retains much of the emphasis medicine places on measurability and objectivity. As discussed in Chapter 5, this stance is not always compatible with the new claims being made for nursing.

For example, the concept of 'care' has long been a central element of nursing. Some would even say that within the health professions, care is unique to nursing. Not surprisingly therefore, recent theory—in a bid to ensure nursing's autonomy—has chosen to retain and develop the caring role of the nurse. The emphasis on care, however, has brought many problems. Nurses have long grappled with what it means to provide *paid* care when care in general is seen as a virtue associated with compassion, patience or even servitude. Care is not generally understood to be a marketable commodity. In addition, we now have to reconcile the notion of tender loving care with the demands of many nursing theorists for scientific measurability and objectivity.

The desire to be scientific has led, by and large, to a romance with the methods of the 'hard' sciences, with a developing preference for analytical skills, theoretical knowledge and quantitative assessment. At the same time practical knowledge, experience and intuition are devalued (Gordon 1986). But not all aspects of nursing are amenable to quantitative analysis. What constitutes 'care' is a good example. I am not suggesting that there should be a complete lack of assessment within nursing, but that a qualitative measure might often be more appropriate. As Steve Wright points out, if we try to define aspects of nursing too carefully we may end up severely confining it instead. By drawing precise boundaries about what is and is not nursing knowledge and practice we may effectively straightjacket the development of nursing. This would be tragic, all the more so if Wright is correct in his suspicions that some theorising is aimed more at enhancing the status of the theorist than serving the interests of nursing itself (1985).

In a similar vein, Kitson (1985) points out that in attempting to be systematic and describe nursing so specifically, the affective relationship between nurse and patient, together with the expectations and limitations of this relationship, are overlooked. In other words, much contemporary nursing theory neglects the more personal and non-measurable aspects of nursing practice. (Nowhere is this more clearly the case than in the field of sexual health care.)

Developments in nursing are largely centred around an upsurge of interest in nursing ideologies and in the creation of new nursing models. There is some confusion, but for the most part, *nursing ideologies* (also known as nursing paradigms) are understood as formal statements of beliefs and values about nursing, society, health, illness and people. These form a basis from which nursing practice can be developed (see, for example, Hunt and Marks-Maran 1986).

This sense of ideology as consciously constructed ideas contrasts with the way it is understood within the social sciences, as largely unconscious, unformulated presuppositions. To avoid confusion, the nursing usage is adopted in this chapter unless specifically stated otherwise. Nonetheless, ideology in the unformulated sense also exists within nursing. Each nurse has a personal ideology, her own beliefs and values shaped by her particular social background, education, religious views, political persuasion etc., of which she may not be fully aware but which will undoubtedly influence her nursing care. Furthermore, the teaching carried out within schools of nursing and the policies of nursing units are informed by both formulated *and* unformulated beliefs and values of staff members (just think of the issue of homosexuality, for example.)

Nursing models act as a framework for the assessment of patients' needs and the planning, giving and evaluation of care. Models suggest ways of putting the nursing process into practice by helping to clarify thought about elements of nursing practice in specific situations and demonstrating the relationships between these elements. There are many different types of nursing models—for example developmental, systems, interactionist or human needs models. However, whichever model is used, it influences the kind of assessment made, the goals of nursing care and how to achieve them; the model lies behind the nurse's thinking at each stage of the nursing process (McFarlane 1986). The choice of one model over another depends not only on the patient's individual circumstances and needs, but also on the extent to which the values and assumptions inherent within the model match those held by the nurse or her nursing team (whichever is responsible for choosing a model). This suggests that both personal and nursing ideologies are to some extent expressed through the nursing model.

Recent trends in nursing theory are thought to bring advantages for patients and for nursing as a whole. They have certainly brought costs which, unfortunately, are often borne by the individual nurse. It has already been stated that the change associated with the introduction of the nursing process—a move from task allocation to patient allocation—has brought the nurse into a more intimate relationship with the patient and therefore subject to increased emotional stress. Similarly, nursing models may help nurses to recognise patients' problems more effectively, but they may nevertheless not h̀ave the resources to cope with the problems they identify. This is most clearly the case when nursing assessment raises the role of social issues such as unemployment or poor housing in the creation of ill health. Because of this, as Kershaw and Salvage (1986) point out, the use of nursing models demands more support and attention to nurse welfare than has previously existed.

This discussion of nursing theory has raised two fundamental points. One is that nursing theory is not built on some kind of ultimate truth, but will shift in emphasis according to the interests of its practitioners and, especially, its leaders; nursing ideology has to be remembered as a set of *beliefs*, not facts. Second, a number of nursing theorists currently place great store on nursing not only as a science but also as a particular type of scientific endeavour. First and foremost they respect the observable, the measurable, the definable. But nursing is as much an art as a science, and its interests and those of its patients are not always best served by the so-called 'hard' sciences. To recognise the value of knowledge based on qualitative as well as quantitative research is to give more positive acknowledgement to the personal element of the nurse-patient relationship.

I do not dispute that it is valuable to have recognisable principles on which to base practice and models through which ideology can be transformed into practice. But the value of these lasts only as long as it is remembered, first, that ideology as a set of ideas is always open to debate and, indeed, must be constantly questioned, and second, that nursing models should be seen primarily as tools by which the nurse can organise her thoughts and subsequently her nursing care; we must guard against the reverse in which the model becomes a straightjacket for the nurse.

Nursing theory and sexuality

Just as there are different levels of nursing theory—the basic concepts (ideologies) and the conceptual tools (models) to carry them into practice—so too are there different levels of problems concerning the way nursing theory deals with sexuality.

At the first level there can be ideological problems. Sexuality may be expressed physically but it is also a theoretical concept; how we interpret sexuality and the sexual health needs of patients depends on how we understand society, what it is to be human and so on. Some of the assumptions, beliefs and values commonly associated with sexuality and detrimental to nursing care have been raised in earlier parts of the book. These may well constitute part of a nurse's personal ideology, be dominant in the training she receives or inherent in the nursing model she chooses. Because of the taboos which surround sexuality, and because it is understood as 'natural', beliefs and assumptions are given little critical examination and come to be accepted as facts. At the same time the information nurses decide to collect in patient assessment and on which nursing care will be based depends, to a large extent, on such unquestioned values. Consequently, so-called 'sexual health care' can be based on prejudices and assumptions which the nurse is allowed to mistake for some kind of ultimate truth.

Second, there can be problems in the relationship between nursing theory and sexuality at the level of the model. Just how useful nursing models are in providing sexual health care depends in part on the choice of model used in any particular situation. Models are not all based on the same values and assumptions about the individual and his or her needs, or the role of nurses. For the sake of brevity I intend to examine only one model in any depth, the Roper/Logan/Tierney model for nursing (or RLT model for short). This model has been described as very close to a medical model in its emphasis on physiological systems (Aggleton and Chalmers 1986) but there are several good reasons for choosing it here. As Pearson says, the RLT model may be applied to all fields of nursing and, as 'the only developed model published by and for British nurses', appears to have a clearer relationship to nursing in this country than other models (1983). Additionally, it is one of the few which specifically refers to sexuality (although other models do not necessarily exclude the consideration of sexuality).

The Roper/Logan/Tierney model

Briefly the RLT model has five components or dimensions, which represent tools or mental aids to help the nurse identify the problems or potential problems of individual patients and to intervene where appropriate (see for example, Roper *et al.* 1985). The model is deliberately uncomplicated. Rather than exhausting every aspect of nursing, it is intended to act as a framework which can help learners think about nursing in general terms. From this they can go on to develop individualised practice.

The RLT model has an implicit ideology. It sees nursing as a link between the technical procedures associated with the treatment of disease and the maintenance of everyday physical and mental functions essential for the patient's comfort and well-being. It also envisages nursing as concerned with 'maintaining health, preventing sickness, enhancing self-help and promoting maximum independence according to the individual person's capacity.' (*ibid*: 3–4). The model is based on a theory of human needs represented by various activities—the *activities of living* (or ALs). These are:

> maintaining a safe environment;
> communicating;
> breathing;
> eating and drinking;
> eliminating;
> personal cleansing and dressing;
> controlling body temperature;
> mobilising;
> working and playing;
> expressing sexuality;
> dying.

Roper and her associates point out that the more the activities of living are analysed, the more complex each one of them appears. For example, each has biological, psychological and social aspects. Furthermore, the ALs are interrelated; to take one example, expressing sexuality cannot be neatly separated from communication. Collectively, these activities form the central focus of the model and are cross-cut by the model's four other dimensions.

Of these, *lifespan* recognises the temporal aspect of each person's life. This dimension acknowledges that the patient is an individual at a particular point in his lifespan between conception and death. That is to say, there is an inherent recognition within the model that a person will undergo change related to age.

Linked to this dimension is another—the concept of a *dependence–independence continuum* in which the patient is recognised as possessing a greater or lesser independence according to his or her stage in the lifespan and the circumstances which may cross-cut this, such as the individual's state of health or environmental factors.

Another dimension of the model, *factors influencing the activities of living*, is concerned with the effects of physical, psychological, socio-cultural, environmental and politic-economic factors on the way the activities of living as basic needs are perceived and met.

The final dimension of the model, which interacts with all the others, is concerned with knowledge of just how and why an individual carries out the activities of living in the way he does. This dimension is termed *individualising nursing*; knowledge of a patient's individuality is seen as a prerequisite for planning individualised nursing care based on the nursing process.

Using this model, nursing care develops from an assessment which identifies the necessity and extent to which nurses should assist the patient in carrying out the activities of living. Assessment involves a consideration of each AL in the context of the other components of the model and the identification of any problems. Nursing intervention may then take many forms, such as the provision of information, material resources, instrumental care or emotional support.

Use of the model

So how useful is this particular model in guiding nursing practice, or more specifically, in incorporating a consideration of the patient's sexuality into the process of nursing? In order to examine the model's usefulness we shall look essentially at the opportunities it allows for assessment and identification of patients' potential or actual problems. Much, of course, depends on how

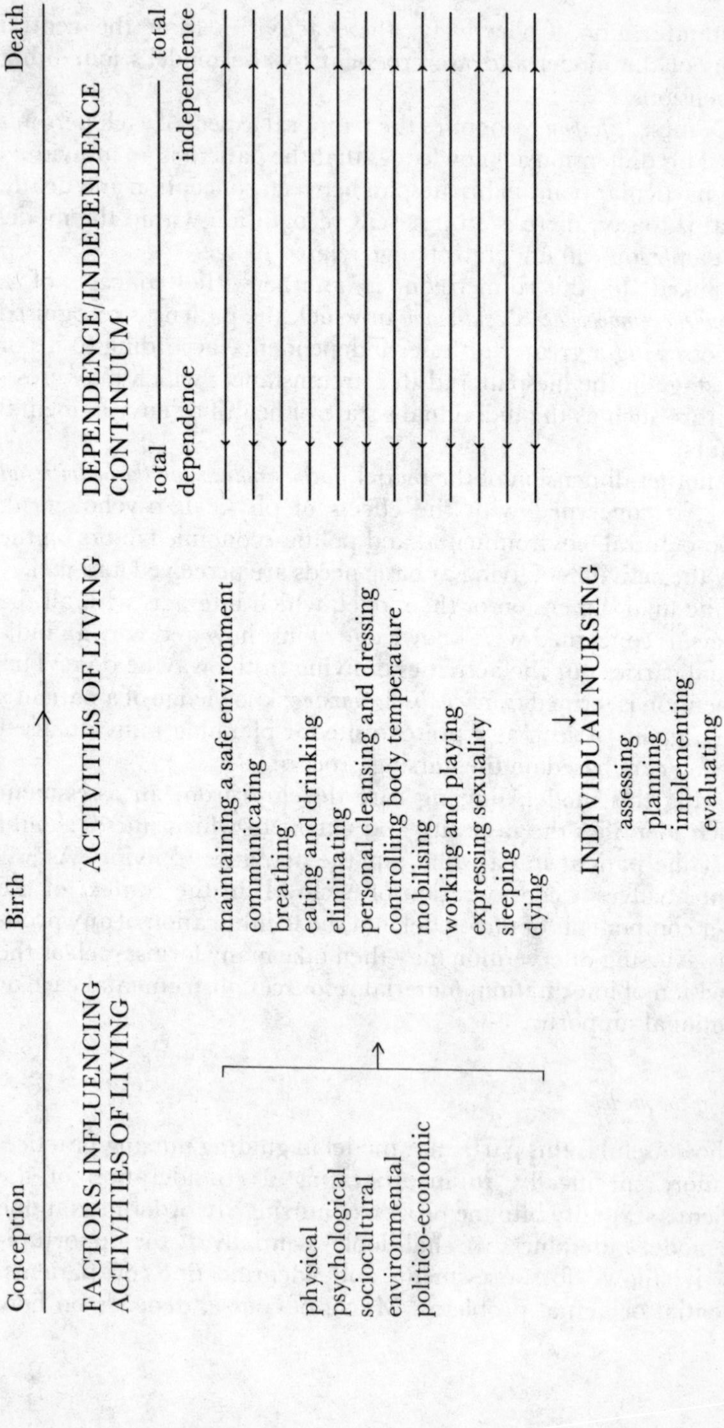

Conception	Birth			Death

LIFESPAN

FACTORS INFLUENCING ACTIVITIES OF LIVING

ACTIVITIES OF LIVING

maintaining a safe environment
communicating
breathing
eating and drinking
eliminating
personal cleansing and dressing
controlling body temperature
mobilising
working and playing
expressing sexuality
sleeping
dying

DEPENDENCE/INDEPENDENCE CONTINUUM

total dependence ——— total independence

physical
psychological
sociocultural
environmental
politico-economic

INDIVIDUAL NURSING

assessing
planning
implementing
evaluating

(Source: Roper *et al* 1985:64)

Figure 3   *Roper, Logan and Tierney model for nursing.*

'expressing sexuality' is interpreted, but this is an ideological problem, and to a certain extent, separate from the question of the model's usefulness in planning sexual health care. Many nurses I spoke to said they did not find the RLT model helpful in this respect. However, on reflection the main problem appeared to be in the way the model was applied, rather than with the model itself.

> 'We use the Roper model of the various activities of daily living. We go through all those and we usually use them quite a lot in class. And *in theory* it's all very good. One of those of course is expressing sexuality and that's important. But when it actually comes to doing it in class, what do you talk about? You talk about helping women to look better after they've had their hysterectomy so their husbands still want to have sex with them. You spend ages on breathing and then you get to the end of the list—you get to dying and expressing sexuality and how we should talk to patients and get them to express their feelings—and that's it! No-one ever does it. We write it in our care plans time and time again: "Encourage questions and help the patient to express their feelings and anxieties about this"—but it's never really. approached.'   (Third-year student)

Within the RLT model, the ALs component as a whole allows for the fact that sexuality touches many aspects of people's lives—so much so that nursing care plans can become fairly repetitive. Webb (1985a) has pointed out that with the RLT model, concern with personal appearance can equally come under the ALs of 'expressing sexuality', 'personal cleansing and hygiene', or 'working and playing'. She claims this is something of a drawback. In order to save repetition, many nurses reserve the AL 'expressing sexuality' to cover those things directly concerned with reproduction (such as menstruation), often reducing sexuality to a purely biological dimension and leaving no space for the consideration of other forms of sexuality, such as erotic sex or body image. If we are to avoid this drawback, repetition seems unavoidable.

The most important point about the RLT model is that to assess sexual health, all dimensions of the model and their inter-relationships must be fully considered. The various stages of this process do not necessarily all need to be documented, and it is therefore not as time-consuming as it may sound. Instead the various dimensions of the model can act as *aides-mémoire*; they provide a framework for how to think about the patient's needs in relation to sexuality which might otherwise be ignored or neglected. The following paragraphs contain examples of ways in which the various dimensions of the model can be drawn on to build an initial picture of the patient's possible needs in relation to sexual health. This picture can then be developed and refined over time by observation, discussion and a few well-considered questions. To clarify my points I take the situation of a hypothetical patient (Linda), a thirty-year-old, unmarried woman with breast cancer who has been admitted to hospital for lumpectomy to be followed by chemotherapy.

Expressing sexuality

First let us consider the AL 'expressing sexuality' and how this may be interpreted. According to the ideology underlying the model, it is a human need to express sexuality and the nurse's task is to assist in this when necessary if this contributes towards health. At the same time nurses should help the patient to be independent of such assistance as soon as possible.

According to Roper and her colleagues, the 'activity of expressing sexuality' appears essentially concerned with the expression of sexual identity (by which they mean being either male or female) through the accessories that characterise men or women, such as style of dress, use of perfume, etc. (*ibid*: 293). In other words, expressing sexuality according to these authors is essentially about expressing gender. Even erotic sex is seen to be little more than a medium for demonstrating masculinity or femininity. Clearly, this is a very narrow understanding of the way in which sexuality can be expressed. We need to broaden our horizons a little, and one way of doing this is to consider the expression of sexuality by looking systematically at the components Roper *et al.* claim for each AL—namely its biological, psychological and social aspects. The biological component of sexuality is often understood to be represented by the physical structures and function of the reproductive system (male and female sex organs, secondary sexual characteristics and the menstrual cycle) together with control of fertility. But, as suggested in Chapter 2, the expression of sexuality concerns the body as a whole: the sense the body has of itself (proprioception),

BIOLOGICAL	PSYCHOSOCIAL
sex organs and secondary sexual characteristics	interpersonal and sexual relationships
menstrual cycle/fertility control	erotic sex/psychosexual response
proprioception	body image
tactile sensation	proxemics (or cultural space)
body products	gender role and identity

Figure 4 *Components of the Activity of Living 'expressing sexuality'.*

the skin that experiences touch (tactile sensation) and the smell and substances that issue from the body (body products).

Because of the nature of sexuality—the way, for example, that sexual preference and behaviour can be socially influenced and yet also a matter of personal choice—the psychological and social components of expressing sexuality are hard to separate out. They will therefore be treated as a single component which includes erotic sex, psychosexual response, sexual and interpersonal relationships, body-image, proxemics, gender role, and gender identity.

Psychosocial component of the AL 'expressing sexuality'

Interpersonal and sexual relationships

Linda is unmarried, but this does not mean she is asexual. Nor can it be assumed she is heterosexual. If she is in a sexual relationship at the moment is it, for example, one that will provide her with support over the course of her treatment? If not, are there others (family, friends) who can offer this? Will the nature of Linda's illness or her hospitalisation change her personal and sexual relationships? How can she be comforted and sustained while in hospital? Does she have sufficient privacy for this?

Erotic sex/psychosexual response

Will breast cancer affect Linda's sense of herself as a sexual person? Does it have any implications for her preferred modes of sexual expression? Will it exacerbate any pre-existing sexual difficulties? How can she be reassured of her continuing sexual attractiveness? How might the effects of surgery, general anaesthesia or chemotherapy affect sexual expressiveness?

Body image

Was Linda satisfied with her breasts (for example their size and shape) before breast cancer was discovered? To what extent is she concerned about her body's appearance in relation to cultural norms? How might breast surgery affect her body image? Will her chemotherapy regime result in hair loss? What does Linda's hair represent to her?

Proxemics

What is Linda's reaction to close contact with hospital staff, to breast examination, to the close proximity of other patients?

Gender role and identity

How does breast cancer/surgery affect the way Linda feels about herself as a woman? In which ways does she usually express her femininity (for example, clothes, social role, employment, aspirations)? Will ill health affect these?

The biological component of the AL 'expressing sexuality'

Sexual organs/secondary sexual characteristics

Have physical characteristics of Linda's breasts (for example small size, drooping shape, 'unusual' hair distribution, inverted nipples) affected Linda's attitude toward her breasts and subsequently to self-examination? Does she know how to do self-examination? How was the breast lump discovered? Is she worried about her future ability to breastfeed?

Menstrual cycle/fertility control

Is Linda concerned that her periods might be disrupted by chemotherapy or that she might be unable to conceive at a later date? Will she need information about contraception to prevent pregnancy during chemotherapy?

Proprioception

Does Linda have a different sense of her breasts because of the presence of malignancy or the intervention of a surgeon?

Tactile sensation

Are Linda's breasts highly sensitive, so causing embarrassment during examination? Otherwise does she find touch reassuring or intrusive?

Body products

Is Linda concerned she might have to use a bedpan? Is she anxious about coping with menstruation while in hospital?

Using these sorts of questions as mental reminders allows nurses over a period of time to build up a basic picture of what expressing sexuality might mean for a particular patient in certain circumstances. This basic picture can then be developed by the introduction of the model's other dimensions.

Lifespan

'Sexual development' is a more obvious example of how lifespan and the expression of sexuality might interact, although as a concept this has its limitations. All too often, for example, sexual development is seen simply in terms of physiological change (such as the development of secondary sexual characteristics) or gender-role conformity (whether, for instance, small girls become interested in playing with dolls). Moreover, awareness that a woman is menopausal is not helpful if it is accompanied by an assumption on the nurse's part that post-menopausal women are asexual.

More usefully the lifespan dimension can prompt the nurse to think about aspects of the patient's sexuality (for example body image, the need for touch, sexual needs and the ability to meet these in the face of physical or mental change) within the context of prevailing social expectations and attitudes towards the sexuality of people of the patient's age group and the extent to which the patient wishes to conform to these.

For example, the assumptions concerning sexuality that might be made about a woman of Linda's age-group are that she is sexually active and fertile, that she is married, planning marriage, or has a steady boyfriend, and that she will want children although she may be leaving it a little late. These *may*, roughly speaking, be Linda's concerns. She may be anxious to have a long-term, committed relationship such as marriage and she may want children. In this case, how does breast cancer affect these aspirations? Does it make them seem more remote as possibilities? Does it make her more anxious about her potential fertility? How does a sense of her potential fertility contribute to the overall sense she has of herself? Is she worried that breast surgery will make her breasts ugly in comparison with those of other women of her age? Linda may have none of these particular concerns—or she may have some and not others. She may, for instance, not wish for a heterosexual relationship, but plans to have children via artificial insemination. If this is the case she may face criticism and pressure from family or friends to conform to their expectations and this pressure may be accentuated in some way by the presence of breast cancer.

Dependence–independence continuum

Looking at the AL 'expressing sexuality' in the light of the dependence–independence continuum helps us to think about the extent to which a patient is physically or emotionally capable of meeting the need to express sexuality. It may mean identifying the way in which the patient is able to deal with changes in sexual behaviour made necessary by illness and what form any help should take. The effects of increased dependency on self-image should also be considered. Although she is unlikely to become more physically dependent on others in order to express herself sexually, in Linda's case the nature of her illness and the anxieties it prompts for the future may make her more *emotionally* dependent on friends or partner, and perhaps more needy of touch. Again, this increased dependency may affect self-image.

Factors influencing the ALs

The dimension of the RLT model 'factors influencing the ALs' can prompt nurses to consider the way in which external influences such as social norms affect the AL 'expressing sexuality'. These influences, for example, may be shaping the patient's attitude to sexuality in the face of physical change. Social norms may affect the extent to which changes in sexual practice or gender role will be viewed as possible. In addition, this dimension of the model can prompt nurses and patients to think about the patient's lifestyle and how, for example, cultural or social values may have contributed to present ill health. An understanding of the way gender role can influence health is valuable here (see pp. 16–17).

In the case of our patient Linda, although it is unlikely that lumpectomy will impose change on her previous sexual behaviour, the fatigue and nausea she may experience with chemotherapy may temporarily affect sexual response and consequently place new demands on Linda and any partner to find other forms of expressiveness. These may be very different from their customary and perhaps more socially-accepted forms of love-making and therefore difficult to initiate. It is also worth considering the effect cultural norms may have on Linda's attitude towards examination by male doctors, intimate procedures by strangers, and the thought of being partially naked in theatre.

Individualising nursing

Finally the dimension known as 'individualising nursing' is used to focus on the uniqueness of the way the patient expresses sexuality and the particular nursing care this suggests. For example, the extent to which women will welcome encouragement to use cosmetics and see this as a sign of recovery will depend on the extent to which they see make-up as an important element of femininity in the first place. In Linda's case, individualised nursing might include the need for:

> space to discuss fears of desertion by any partner;
> privacy during partner's visits;
> information about anatomy and physiology of breast in relation to effects of surgery and chemotherapy on breastfeeding;
> a discussion of breast appearance in relation to cultural norms.

From these examples we can see how the RLT model is potentially useful in assessing the patient's needs: 'potentially', because a great deal hinges both on the way in which 'sexuality' is interpreted and that all the various dimensions of the model are applied (even where this involves a certain amount of repetition). All too often in practice however, if sexuality is given any consideration at all, it is only under the ALs dimension. In other words, there is a failure by nurses to use the model properly and to exploit its strongest point—its multi-dimensional nature. As a result, in many patient assessments (formal or informal), the expression of sexuality is given scant attention.

Identification of nursing goals

As suggested earlier, using a sophisticated model can be something of an empty exercise if the ideology on which it rests is inadequate. The absence of clearly stated beliefs and values about sexuality can mean the nurse is unclear as to what she is assessing and why. In addition to this it is, curiously, quite possible for the patient's needs to be accurately assessed while nursing goals miss the point entirely.

For example, Roper and others (*ibid*) have provided examples of the problems which might be identified within the AL 'expressing sexuality' and the nursing goals associated with this. They suggest, for instance, that a patient's assessment may reveal that institutionalisation is imposing restrictions on the opportunity to be sexually expressive. The nursing goals arising from this include minimising the disruption of sexual expression while institutionalised. But let us think about 'sexual expression' and what it means. Despite increasingly varied interpretations of this term by nurses, there is rarely any explicitly stated belief shaping nursing practice which advocates the patient's right to *erotic* sexual expressiveness—at least *while still a patient*. Even Roper *et al*. suggest the patient should be allowed to go home 'where appropriate' so that sexual relationships can be maintained. The assumption is that there is no place for sexual expressiveness of the erotic kind within hospitals or other institutions. But of course some patients cannot go home. As one nurse said to me:

'For those people having long-term care, for instance those with mental illness or cancer, we very often chop off half their life.

Then we wonder why marriages fail for cancer patients! And it is basically the health care provider that does this. Instead of encouraging people to carry on with their normal sexual practices . . . we say "You've got to take a break in your life now and you can't start again until we say you can"—without considering what we're doing to the person, to the relationship and to both people's long-term future. Because basically physical contact is thought dirty in the health-care system and the attitude is "We're not having any of that under our roof"!'

(Nurse Adviser, RCN Oncology Society)

This trend is partly due to practical problems, such as the provision of privacy described in Chapter 7. However it is also a matter of interpretation and the way in which the concept of sexuality is being put across in nurse training. I have already pointed out the apparent narrowness of Roper's interpretation. Of course sexuality has many dimensions and sexual expressiveness does not necessarily mean sexual intercourse, masturbation or other forms of erotic sex. Nonetheless, for some patients the issue of the maintainance of sexual relationships involving some level of eroticism still has to be faced.

At the moment this issue is largely being evaded because of a tendency within nursing and nurse education to turn old assumptions inside out, and to interpret sexuality as *predominantly* non-physical and non-erotic. This trend has been partly prompted by a desire to overturn older and equally limiting views of sexuality in which it was assumed to mean just penetrative sex. At the same time it is also a convenient way of dodging the practical problems that arise with any acknowledgement of the patient's erotic sexuality. This means that while the expression of sexuality is recognised as an important AL, there is a preference for understanding the sexuality referred to *primarily* as gender. As a result, the nurse in training is generally taught to consider the patient's expression of sexuality either as the expression of femininity in the case of a woman (for example, by the use of make-up or a frilly nightdress) or with a male patient, the demonstration of masculinity by the use of aftershave etc. Put another way, nurse teachers promote an understanding of the expression of sexuality as synonymous with an attractiveness defined by gender stereotypes.

Clearly, for many people toiletries, cosmetics, clothes and so on do play a significant part in providing a sense of identity. They may be especially important for those whose morale has been seriously undermined by ill health. But these gestures have to be recognised as part of gender identity, and only a small component of sexual identity. The danger of missing this point is that emphasis on the expression of gender takes the nurse's attention away from other less gender-specific elements of sexuality. The term 'sexuality' covers many things, including sensuality, eroticism, libido, sexual fulfilment, warmth, power, and tenderness and in considering the patient's expression of sexuality we should be thinking of all these as much as gender.

Challenging gender stereotypes

This is not to say that nurses should ignore the issue of gender. Earlier on I mentioned the impact of gender role on health—very briefly, that social expectations of men and women constitute specific forms of stress which are currently expressed, for example, in a higher rate of heart disease among men and of mental disorders among women. What will be suggested here is that where nurses recognise that gender-role expectations are contributing towards ill health or poor recovery, part of their nursing care must include the provision of information and support for the patients which will help them challenge these expectations.

There are already moves in this direction by some nurses but, by and large, they do not go far enough. Webb (1985a) for instance gives attention to the important role of gender in an example of the way Roy's Adaptation model can be used to incorporate sexuality into nursing care. As she points out, this model does not specifically refer to sexuality, although it does allow it to be incorporated into nursing care as elements of its various subsystems. In Webb's example, her patient is a taxi-driver recovering from a myocardial infarction. The Roy model was chosen as a basis for planning nursing care because of the patient's need to introduce changes into his life to regain health and prevent a further heart attack. His sedentary occupation, obesity and poor eating habits, together with stress arising from his association of masculinity with the responsibility of 'bread-winning' are all seen as having a possible causal role in his illness.

Using this model, Webb shows how the influence of cultural values such as gender can be borne in mind throughout the nursing assessment. For example, she identifies a relationship between the patient's obesity and the lack of knowledge men in general have about cooking and food values. She sees a further connection between the patient's obesity (in the sense of 'being big') and masculinity. She also makes a link between the patient's concern that his sex life may be at an end because of illness and the extent to which cultural stereotypes of sexuality and gender promote this concern.

One aim in drawing up a teaching plan for this patient is to instruct him that sex is not a particularly strenuous activity, and, for example, that once he can climb two flights of stairs he is fit enough to engage in sexual activity. Factually there is nothing wrong with this information—as far as it goes. What seems strange, though, is that recognition is given to the influence of cultural values (in the form of gender-role expectations) upon health status, yet nursing intervention makes no attempt to deal with this. The patient will therefore probably continue unquestioningly to associate masculinity with making financial provision for his family, and will no doubt continue to link 'manliness' with some sexual activities rather than others. But what if he is unable to return to work, or remains unable to climb two flights of stairs? Is he no longer a man? Does he lose all chance of sexual expressiveness? Of course not; other less strenuous options remain open to him, although it is unlikely he will feel confident to consider adopting these unless he has come to terms with the contradictions in gender role that they represent.

What is wrong with Webb's plan for patient care is that not enough is being done with much of the valuable information gathered in the original nursing assessment. And, as Hunt and Marks-Maran say, gathering personal information is an invasion of privacy if it is not for planning and giving nursing care (1986). If cultural values such as those associated with gender are identified as influencing health, they cannot be ignored. Therefore in addition to the information Webb's plan provides, it is a crucial part of nursing care to discuss the limitations imposed by gender role and, if necessary, encourage the patient to challenge these and explore alternatives. As Chapman has said, nursing can act as a mechanism for change and the nurse is in a unique position to influence patients (1978).

This chapter has looked at the way nursing theory attempts to deal with the patient's sexuality. Using the example of the RLT model it finds the model itself has great potential in aiding nurses to assess the patient's sexual health *providing* it is the right choice of model for a given situation and that all the dimensions of the model are fully employed. Much also depends on the ideology underlying such models if they are to be successfully applied. One major area of concern in terms of ideology is that there is generally a limited understanding of gender and sexuality. The two concepts are often confused, frequently with untoward emphasis on gender. Moreover, gender stereotypes are taken as given and are not open to questioning. This has serious implications for nursing assessment and care.

Each nursing unit, whether at ward, hospital or district level, should clarify the ideology in which nursing care will be rooted by identifying its beliefs and values about nursing, sexuality and sexual health. In·addition, there should be greater openness to discussion within each unit, so that if basic policy towards sexuality is developed by the more senior nurses it can still be challenged by any individual nurse, should she feel it necessary. A specific policy might be developed collectively by clinical nurses, closely attuned to their understanding of their patients' needs, instead of being developed by those whose involvement is rather more remote. In either case, all nurses need to be able clearly to identify, discuss and question the beliefs and values concerning sexuality which ultimately determine this aspect of nursing care. As part of this process nurse education should provide a broader understanding of the issues involved in any consideration of sexuality and gender. Suggestions concerning nurse education are included in the final chapter.

Further reading

Pearson A., Vaughan B. (1986). *Nursing Models for Practice*. London: Heinemann.

9

The nurse and sexual health care

Introduction

In previous chapters we have looked at a number of the problems that prevent concern for the patient's sexual health being translated into actual care. First there are conceptual problems, either in understanding the multi-dimensional nature of sexuality or in the use of nursing models to plan sexual health care. Second, there are practical problems. Sexuality in one or other of its various forms plays an important role *within* nursing, shaping its development, its aspirations, its knowledge base, and especially, the nurse–patient relationship. The effects of sexuality on the structure and process of nursing can seriously affect patient care.

Throughout the book suggestions have been made about how these problems might be dealt with. Broadly speaking, they fall into two groups. One is concerned with improvements in the education of nurses (or, in some instances, the education of other health workers). Suggestions in the second group deal with the support that should be available to nurses who are concerned with sexual health care. However, in order to look in more detail at the kind of training and support that should be provided, some clarification of an appropriate role for the nurse in sexual health care is needed.

Sexual health care and the role of the nurse

What do we expect of the nurse when we speak of the provision of sexual health care? Following what has been said in earlier chapters, sexual health care might reasonably be seen as a vital element of care for *any* patient. However it will not be important in the same way for each patient. For example, sexual health care will be of particular significance for those experiencing irreversible anatomical or physiological change as with hysterectomy, emphysema, or arthritis. But care of the sexual aspect of the patient is often important even where there is no obvious challenge to the patient's sexuality; the mere process of becoming a patient has implications for sexuality by affecting self-concept. Moreover, sexual problems (that is, sexual dysfunction) may be precipitated or made worse by ill health. The issues with which sexual health care might concern itself are therefore wide-ranging. Should the general nurse be expected to deal with all these and acquire all the many different skills they demand? I think not. While some of the patient's concerns about sexuality are best dealt with by the general nurse, there are others which are more appropriately dealt with by specialists.

Basic sexual health care

Among health workers, nurses are in a unique position to assess sexual health because of their involvement in the physical care of patients, including round-the-clock contact, and their opportunities to meet patients' friends and families (Miller 1984). Because of their opportunity to offer sexual health care, all nurses should have an understanding of the many dimensions of sexuality and some awareness of how these may affect the patient and his or her care. Nursing responsibility in sexual health care should extend to all patients, regardless of their principal nursing or medical diagnosis. This responsibility involves an understanding of gender role and of the link between gender expectations and ill health. It also includes a recognition of the significance of body-boundary and body products, the way self-concept can be affected by ill-health, and the subtleties of the nurse-patient relationship. This level of awareness then has to be translated into nursing care.

As with any other focus of nursing care, areas of concern can be identified during nurse assessment—especially if this is built up over time. Nursing intervention at a basic level of sexual health care may take the form of identifying a specific problem in collaboration with the patient and helping him or her to resolve the problem, either by the provisions of information or by making the appropriate referral.

The identification of problems by nurses raises the issue of whether or not they should take a specific sexual history as part of patient assessment. In the United States the nurse is expected to ask patients a series of formalised questions as a matter of routine. Kneisl and Wilson (1984) suggest enquiries such as 'How important has sexual activity been in your life?' 'What does sexuality mean to you?', or 'How are your needs for intimacy being met?'

These are very personal and probing questions, which some people will resent deeply. They are also rather like asking 'How long is a piece of string?'; it is doubtful whether many people would be able to put a reply into words, even if they wanted to. And even if the patient genuinely attempts to answer these sorts of questions, what does such knowledge of the patient achieve? Probably very little—at least while current constraints such as inadequate training, understaffing and lack of support limit the way in which nurses can handle such information.

Woods (1984) claims that taking a sexual history is useful simply for its inherent therapeutic value, providing patients with the opportunity to talk about their concerns. She suggests a very brief sexual history can be incorporated into a more general history and can consist, for example, of the following questions:

1. Has anything (such as illness or pregnancy) changed the way you feel about yourself as (a woman, mother, man, father)?
2. Has anything (for example disease, surgery) affected your sex life?

Alternatively the nurse can form her assessment by informal means, free from the limitations imposed by pieces of paper, standardised lists or formal interviews:

'I have always taught the nursing process on the basis of the activities of living and ... by talking to patients. It's not just a piece of paper that you have to complete in four hours; it's actually a patient profile that you can get together in forty-eight hours just by being with the patient and talking to them—getting to know them and picking up their cues. And there are all sorts of cues you can pick up if you're listening. The pieces of paper tend to stop you from listening. And they're also attempts to stop the patient from talking, because they're not sure how much you're going to write down and who else is going to see it. But if you take a patient profile just in conversation and then record your thoughts later—then you've got a model of care.'

(Nurse tutor)

This method seems all the more valuable for dealing with the specific issue of sexual health.

Whether a formal or informal approach is adopted, once a problem concerning sexual health is revealed, it is important to elicit a description of the problem in the patient's own terms, an understanding of the patient's concept of the cause of the problem and a clear picture of the patient's expectations or goals. This last point is particularly important in deciding whether or not the nurse should refer a patient to a specialist (Woods *ibid*).

Clearly, assessment is more difficult in some situations, such as day care. In the case of hospital day-patients, assessment and the implementation of care can begin prior to admission with the involvement of out-patient nurses. They may provide the patient with information about his admission and the nature of any procedure involved, and may allow the patient the opportunity to discuss any fears he or she may have. This pre-admission care already exists in some places for particular patients (for example, those booked for termination of pregnancy). It could, however, be extended to many more, and be far more conscious of sexual health concerns—for example, patients for endoscopic investigation may need to discuss the sense of violation they fear the procedure will involve. This kind of care can also be provided by community staff such as practice nurses. However it requires closer liaison than is often found at the moment between nurses working in different areas.

Finally in terms of basic sexual health care, it should be remembered that verbal intervention, whether in the form of a sexual history or the provision of information, is not always sufficient. Indeed in some contexts it may be quite inappropriate, for example, in situations where the nurse violates the patient's body-boundary by the use of instrumental touch or has to deal with the patient's body products. Verbally acknowledging the significance of such acts can make a meal of things and runs the risk of further embarrassing both nurse and patient. Instead, nurses can minimise the threat their actions represent by their manner, by the way in which they use touch or their tone of voice. However this kind of non-verbal intervention often requires more than an intuitive grasp of what is appropriate. Nurses should therefore be encouraged to become more aware of unspoken communication, such as body language, and how to make effective use of it, and more attention must be given to ways in which nurses can demonstrate the non-sexual nature of intimate procedures and how they can 'qualify' apparently seductive behaviour from patients.

Sexual adjustment

In addition to basic sexual health care, nurses have an obligation to help those patients who undergo bodily change to re-establish themselves as confident individuals who are as sexually active as they wish to be. As MacRae and Henderson (1975) have stated, in order to meet this obligation, nurses need to become more competent at including sexual adjustment into patients' overall care plans. Nurses should not, of course, become sex counsellors, but they should become more knowledgeable about sexuality so they can support those patients who, because of changes in health status, wish to explore alternatives to their previous form of sexual expression.

This means that all general nurses must be prepared to deal with this issue *at some level*. But as MacRae and Henderson rightly point out, no-one should *have* to discuss sex. However it remains the nurse's obligation to make it clear to patients that they can initiate discussion on this subject with members of the nursing staff in general. If a nurse recognises that the patient wants to talk about sexual adjustment yet feels uncomfortable about dealing with this issue in person, it is his or her responsibility to involve other members of the health care team who feel more capable of helping.

Certain precautions should be followed by nurses who *do* become involved in this form of care. The patient's moral, religious and personal views should be respected. The nurse's own morality and personal taboos should not be transmitted to the patient. Encouragement about a patient's future ability for sexual expression should not be over-enthusiastic; high expectations may ultimately undermine the patient's confidence if they turn out to be unrealistic. Moreover, counselling should not take place without awareness that changes in sexual practice or role are generally difficult to undertake and may even be threatening to the individual. Possible changes should therefore only be discussed sensitively and realistically and within the context of any relationship the patient may have. The difficulties of partners should also be recognised; they may experience problems with a change of sexual role or if conflicting demands are made of them—for example to act as lover *and* bronchial hygienist for a partner with emphysema (MacRae and Henderson *ibid*).

Nurses should also be prepared to admit when they have insufficient knowledge to deal with a patient's enquiries. Once again they have a responsibility either to find the relevant information or to refer the patient to someone who is better informed. Nurses working within particular specialities, such as coronary care units or wards where post-coronary patients may be transferred prior to discharge, should make it their business to read the literature which exists on the potential problems raised by ischaemic heart disease concerning sexual expression. They should also learn directly from their patients what difficulties they foresee and their priorities, hopes and fears concerning sexuality. Nurses who have experience of helping patients with sexual adjustment should also publish information so that it becomes available to others. This information would clearly be all the more valuable if it was published in collaboration with the patients from whom they have learnt.

In helping with sexual adjustment, the nurse's role is primarily supportive and informative. With suitable training nurses may provide information about the effects of treatment or disease on sexual expression and the alternative forms of expressiveness that remain possible. By doing so they may also give the patient 'permission' to explore alternatives he or she might otherwise regard as taboo. At the same time nurses can help the patient come to terms with changes in self-concept by discussing the social influences on sexuality which indicate its flexibility.

However, knowledge that change is possible is not in itself enough to bring change. Some sexual adjustment will involve major behavioural change such as a shift from a form of lovemaking focused on penetration to non-penetrative sex, or a different sexual role (such as greater passivity), which conflicts with gender identity. Where such significant behavioural change is involved the patient may well need specialised care. In this instance the nurse acts as a screening agent, ideally discussing the issue with members of the health care team and making the appropriate referral. Referral by nurses is a contentious point.

Some doctors, for instance, feel that nurse-initiated referrals to other professionals should be subject to 'scrutiny and agreement' by medical staff (see Mitchell 1984). But there is nothing to suggest that the majority of doctors know anything more about sexuality or sexual problems than most nurses. Indeed Masters (of Masters and Johnson fame) has suggested doctors know no more about the subject than other college graduates and share most of the common misconceptions and taboos of their peers (cited by Fontaine 1976).

In an ideal world, referral would arise from a decision made by a team of doctors, nurses and other health workers. In the absence of this possibility there is no reason why well-informed nurses cannot initiate referrals related to sexual health. Depending on the problem, these may be made to psychosexual counsellors, more general behaviour therapists, to associations (such as SPOD or the Mastectomy Association) or to self-help groups which have special knowledge or experience of the patient's problem.

Psychosexual problems

Sexual dysfunction can happen to anyone and is not restricted to those whose sexual identity is challenged by ill health. Nonetheless it should be borne in mind that patients may well develop psychosexual problems following hospitalisation, disease, treatment or disability. If this is the case they should be offered the opportunity of consulting specialised therapists. Some nurses with a special interest in these problems undertake the training which allows them to work in this field. The general nurse is more concerned with discussing patients' fears and with providing the kind of information they might need to *avoid* the development of psychosexual problems. As we saw earlier, the man who has had a coronary thrombosis may well be concerned that sexual activity will cause further damage to his heart. Without adequate information he may develop impotence or premature ejaculation because of his fear. Suggestions concerning alternative sexual practices and positions which are less physically demanding and the 'permission' to try these are valuable contributions that can be made by the general nurse.

Some patients' psychosexual problems pre-exist their illness. These the general nurse cannot cope with directly. However he or she is in a strong position to increase the patient's self-confidence about sexuality, and indirectly to help the patient cope with such problems. For example, the nurse who discovers a patient has vaginismus when attempting to take a high vaginal swab or cervical smear may be able to use the occasion to dispel some of the fears the patient may have about her own body. She can be reassured that the problem is a relatively common one and does not usually indicate any vaginal abnormality. The nurse *may* be able to help the patient relax sufficiently for examination to be possible and to use this opportunity to indicate that there is nothing unpleasant or dirty about this part of the patient's body. If it appears appropriate, the nurse can encourage the patient to examine herself in an effort to come to terms with her anatomy. In this sort of way nurses can make an appreciable difference to a patient's confidence and self-image. In addition they can discuss the long-term help that is available, indicating what such therapy might involve and making a referral if this is desired.

In summary then, the role of the nurse in sexual health care varies according to the nature of any problem. First there is a basic level of care concerned essentially with non-erotic sexuality; all nurses have a responsibility to provide this level of care. Second, the nurse can play a valuable role in helping the patient adjust to sexual change following ill health. All nurses should be aware of the potential needs of patients undergoing change but not all will feel confident to cope with this dimension of care. They do, however, have a responsibility to find someone who is. Those nurses who are interested in this area should also be able to recognise when the task is beyond their training and referral is necessary. Third, general nurses have a role in recognising ways in which psychosexual problems may be precipitated by ill health. They may also be able to reduce sexual fears by the way they deal with the patient's body. They should have some understanding of what psychosexual treatment involves in order to be able to recognise when referral is appropriate and to discuss with patients what such treatment might involve. All these aspects of the nurse's role in sexual health care have implications for training.

Sexuality and the education debate

Nurses need to be provided with an understanding of sexuality in its fullest sense and its susceptibility to social, cultural and psychological influences. They also need to be aware of ways in which

Traditional practice	Nursing process
Nursing's deference to medicine	Nursing's autonomy
Nursing as a practical activity with the nurse as technician	Nursing as an intellectual activity with the nurse as creative thinker
Nurse passively receives information	Nurse actively seeks information
Nursing role restricted to physical considerations	Nursing role expanded to include behavioural and social considerations
Patient as passive receiver of care	Patient as active participant in care
Diffuse accountability through nursing hierarchy	Individual accountability for nurse

(Adapted from Hollingsworth 1985.)

Figure 5   *Differences between traditional practice and the nursing process.*

these same factors may influence the process of nursing. In Chapter 8 it was suggested that nurses need to be equipped and encouraged to challenge their nursing unit's formulated or unformulated ideology concerning sexuality. This calls for a different educational approach from that presently followed within most schools of nursing, but one that seems possible because of more general changes in thinking about nurse education.

The introduction of the nursing process has enormous implications, not only for the very nature of nursing but also for its educational basis. Figure 5 demonstrates some of the differences between 'traditional' nursing practice and that based on the nursing process. The very different philosophy underlying the nursing process means that nurse education has to equip nurses to think for themselves. This is arguably the direct opposite of the premise on which the traditional approach rested, namely 'If you wanted to think you shouldn't have come into nursing' (see Salvage 1985: 59). Nurses are now being asked to become problem solvers. However they will not become *effective* problem solvers unless they are encouraged to develop a broad framework of knowledge within which free thinking can take place. Nurse education therefore needs to promote understanding and the ability to *use* knowledge rather than learning by rote. Moreover, just as acknowledgement of the patient's right to participate in decision-making is changing the nature of the nurse-patient relationship, the increased accountability expected of individual nurses argues for a similar shift in the relationship between trainees and teachers, nurses and managers. Tutors and managers should be supportive rather than directive.

The use of nursing models also has implications for nurse education. As Wright says: 'A nursing model which focuses solely on the patient and neglects or underestimates the nurses themselves and the social backcloth of the hospital and community is of little value' (1986:40). This suggests that in addition to subjects such as anatomy and physiology, basic training must include not only broad clinical experience but also academic study in the social sciences if it is to expand the trainee's horizons. Recent theoretical developments indicate that nurses should be allowed to be creative and imaginative, and that this requires a broad education which permits them to make decisions in a variety of situations. This point is not particularly new (see, for example Holder 1973, Chapman 1978). However, recent appraisals of nurse education, such as those by the UKCC or the RCN Commission, add their weight to earlier arguments and press for fundamental educational reform. The Commission on Nursing Education recognises the right of the nurse trainee to genuine student status and the right 'to question as well as obey, to discover as well as to be taught, to learn from those who have never been nurses as well as those who have been excellent ones.' (1985:12). Hopefully then, help is at hand as the changes in nurse education which *may* result from these reports would begin to create the sort of intellectual environment conducive to the provision of adequate sexual health care. (The necesary emotional environment is discussed under the heading of 'Support'.)

What also needs to change at an intellectual level, however, is the very knowledge base of nursing. Nursing needs to re-examine the principles on which it is based. Hand in hand with the nursing process and the desire for nursing's autonomy has come an emphasis on quantitative research. Yet as we have seen, the affective relationship between nurse and patient which is so integral to nursing care cannot be quantified. It can, however, be described and learned from if we are less concerned with adopting the criteria on which medical research by and large depends. Nurse education needs to recognise and encourage qualitative as well as quantitative research if we are really going to incorporate an understanding of sexuality into nursing.

Sexuality and nurse tutors

Sexuality and the proper provision of sexual health care by nurses poses certain problems for nurse tutors. To begin with, many are ill-prepared to teach this topic. An American study (Fontaine *ibid*) found that most nurse educators interviewed thought they had a better understanding of sexuality than their students and believed themselves adequately prepared to deal with the subject. Fontaine suspected that this apparent confidence only indicated the educators' lack of understanding of the issues involved, as their own training had made absolutely no reference to sexuality. Moreover, those instructors who professed to recognise the sexual concerns of patients did not suggest to trainees that these might be an issue in any nursing assessment. Fontaine concludes that even the people who are aware of the problem do not always try to do anything about it because of the difficulty people have in discussing sexuality (1976).

The same is probably true in the United Kingdom (see, for example, Webb 1985b). This was certainly indicated by many of the nurses I interviewed, who expressed concern about their tutors' attitudes or abilities to cope with the issues of sexuality. Some were embarrassed by their tutors' obvious difficulties in dealing with sexuality. Others felt their tutors had a poor theoretical grasp of the concepts involved, implying, for example, that sexuality and gender are synonymous. A further group felt resentful that tutors assumed all their trainees would be heterosexual.

While lack of adequate preparation is one concern, it is not necessarily the case that nurse tutors are anyway the best people to teach trainee nurses about sexuality. My own impression is that tutors find the issue extremely difficult to cope with. Not only are they inadequately trained, but a greater emphasis on discussion and a less didactic approach almost inevitably leads to a certain amount of self-disclosure on the part of participants. Jourard (1971) has noted how those who are prepared to disclose information about themselves will establish better communication with those they are trying to reach. Even if self-disclosure is not overt, a good discussion will indirectly reveal some of the attitudes of its participants. Many nurse tutors will find it difficult to combine this role with other aspects of their work and with their overall relationships with trainees. From the perspective of the nurse in training, tutors (and ward staff) may not be ideal people with whom to discuss some aspects of sexuality. Because of a continual awareness of being assessed, trainees are reluctant to have discussions with tutors which may indicate their own doubts and prejudices or even their sexual preferences.

This suggests that at least until there is a change in the present system of training and nurse assessment, courses on human sexuality may be facilitated by nurse tutors but should largely be introduced into the curriculum by others outside the school of nursing. A report on the teaching of sexuality to health workers commissioned by the WHO sees quite positive reasons why material on sexuality is best provided in this way. By involving a number of teachers from different disciplines but working as a team,

> 'material drawn from many sources can be presented within the context of a broad philosophy of human sexuality that gives it coherence and gathers the many pieces, as in a jigsaw puzzle, into an intelligible whole.' (Mace *et al.* 1974:24)

This would not prevent comparatively straightforward information, such as the effects of certain diseases and treatments on sexuality, being incorporated into other parts of the curriculum by tutors.

The danger of this suggestion is that, to some extent, it continues to treat sexuality as something different, special or even suspect because it cannot be dealt with within the normal framework of training. This is a risk but the alternative is to continue as before or to postpone change until the whole system of nurse and tutor training has changed. This could mean a long wait.

The role of nurse tutors

The nurse tutor is ideally placed to portray a positive image of nurses and nursing for nurses and other health workers. This needs to be done quite explicitly, by describing and challenging common images of nurses. In addition, nurse tutors should present trainees with a strong sense of their role—especially in relation to doctors. The notion of the nurse as colleague (as opposed to handmaiden) should be implicit in all their teaching. Too often nurses receive conflicting messages about their position *vis-à-vis* doctors. They are led to believe they have a valuable and autonomous role but their experience tells them they are expected to defer to doctors. The supremacy of medicine has been inferred, for example, by the premium that is placed on lectures given by doctors, even though most doctors have little understanding of the nature of nursing.

Nurse tutors should therefore evaluate their teaching programmes and, where any session is still given over to doctors, question the necessity of instruction by medical staff. Clearly nursing does not wish to isolate itself from the views of other health workers. But sessions which present material based on a medical model as an unquestioned basis for nursing practice are of little value. At the same time, nurse tutors are perhaps best placed among nurses to press for space within the medical curriculum in an attempt to impart an understanding of nursing to medical students. Without a properly informed medical profession there will always be conflict within the nurse-doctor relationship.

Support

Nurses need support over a number of issues which have some bearing on the provision of sexual health care. As stated earlier, the use of the nursing process has made for a greater intimacy between nurse and patient. Moreover, recognition of the patient's right actively to participate in his or her care challenges the traditional relationship between nurse and patient arising from the patient's enforced dependency. These changes may benefit the patient but they also increase the emotional stress to which nurses are subject. There is resentment that there has been no increase in terms of management support to match this. It has also been noted that the clearer identification of patients' problems resulting from the use of nursing models has demonstrated the limitations of nursing. When nurses find themselves unable to meet the problems they have so carefully identified with the patient—

either because of lack of resources, apparently personal short-comings, or the social nature of the problem—they feel they are failing in their nursing care. As Kershaw and Salvage suggest:

> 'The use of models may well require much greater attention being paid to the nurse's welfare and the support she needs to carry out a demanding care programme—not only in terms of staffing levels but in terms of her own psychological needs.'
>
> (*ibid:xiii*)

One of the things I found emerged clearly from talking to trainee nurses was the lack of support they experienced, both generally and in relation to sexuality. Speaking generally, Tschudin (1985) states that nurses should be able to receive support from a number of sources. One way is through an education which includes the psychological aspects of care and the skills of interpersonal communication. Second, occupational health departments should offer physical and emotional help or referral. Counselling services such as the RCN's CHAT should be better advertised. Finally there should be more formal support groups where nurses can 'let off steam' and *receive* care.

Nurses may, however, be reluctant to turn to these modes of support when struggling with issues of sexuality, requiring something more specific. For example, ward-based support groups were available to some of the nurses I spoke with but were often found unsatisfactory. One reason was that little importance was given to these sessions by permanent ward staff: trainee nurses could only attend them if they went instead of taking their tea break. Nurses in some instances found it distressing to discuss problems they were experiencing only to return to them immediately afterwards with nothing really changed. There was no attempt to continue support beyond the confines of the meeting. Therefore instead of feeling in any way 'better' after the support group they felt they had only made themselves more vulnerable by revealing their feelings. Moreover, the ethos of coping come hell or high water, and the background awareness of continual assessment, made it difficult to speak openly.

What might be more effective for coping with sexuality and other emotive issues is a long-term support group composed of nurses of similar experience which runs throughout nurse training. Although these should be quite independent from the school of nursing, it could still be the school's responsibility to ensure that nurses think about such groups when they start training and perhaps give initial guidance in how to set up and run them. These would exist in addition to other forms of support nurses could seek, for example from trained staff counsellors or chaplains. Autonomous support groups could be given recognition through the allocation of time for group work when students are in school, and special study days could be facilitated by the school for a number of such groups, in response to the needs these groups identify. The school could perhaps organise invited speakers and arrange time within the programme for groups to have separate discussions which integrate with their long-term work. In the words of one of the nurses I spoke to:

> 'We need support. I mean there aren't any answers really at the end of the day; you've just got to sort out your own level, what sort of situations you find acceptable and what you don't. But we need support to do it and to know that other people are experiencing similar things.'

A plea for realism

One thing that trainees and others experience in isolation is that many expectations of nurses are quite unrealistic. Farabaugh (1984) has noted that nurse tutors often subject trainees to considerable stress by presenting them with unrealistic portrayals of nurses to emulate, so pushing them to attempt an idealised and unattainable standard of care. One example of this concerns nurses' capacity to deal with their own sexuality.

Many writers have stressed that in order for nurses to be able to include the expression of sexuality and sexual adjustment into a patient's overall care, nurses must first come to terms with their own sexuality. This must be the case—up to a point. Certainly nurses can and should be aware of the effects of social and cultural influences on their individual sexuality and of their personal values and attitudes. But to assume that anyone entirely comes to terms with their sexuality is unrealistic. Many of those who go into nursing have had little chance to develop their own sexual identity before doing so, and of course sexuality is not static, but changes throughout life. On top of this, it is difficult to feel comfortable with one's sexuality when it is constantly being denigrated by some of the unpleasant social attitudes held towards nurses as a group or women in general.

According to one writer, those nurses who are comfortable with their own sexuality and the sexuality of others, who have a thorough understanding of sexual health and who possess or strive towards sensitive communication skills, can integrate sexuality into the nursing process (Lion 1982). But what about the rest of us? Who can truthfully place their hand on their heart and say they are completely at ease—not only with their own—but with everyone else's sexuality? What about the sexuality of the rapist, the sadist, the paedophile or even the Don Juan? Perhaps, to be fair, the author was referring to some kind of 'normal' sexuality we can be comfortable with—but what is normal and who defines it? Looking just at erotic sexuality, for example, if we take hetero-sexual, penile-vaginal intercourse in the 'missionary' position by a naked, married couple twice a week in bed with the lights off as normal, this definition would most probably identify the majority of readers of this book as deviant in one way or another.

A great deal of the nursing literature, although very sensitive in its concern for the patient, gives the dangerous impression that there are significant numbers of nurses who are completely at ease with the issue of sexuality and its integration into nursing. The risk of this is that the rest feel only more inadequate and inept. It suggests that until you feel confident about sexuality in all its aspects you cannot begin to deal with it as a nurse.

In reality it is only through struggling to incorporate sexuality *amid* all our doubts and feelings of inadequacy that we will begin to learn about ourselves and our patients and grow in confidence. Whether it is possible to attain a state of grace and ever come to deal with sexuality in a dispassionate way seems doubtful. I do not even know that this is a worthy goal. After all, if we become glib about sexuality, can we still empathise with most patients' unease? Once sexuality stops being a highly charged issue, what will be left? Unless we continue to recognise the special nature of sexuality, with all the continuing awkwardness that accompanies such an acknowledgement, it seems unlikely that nurses *will* be able to communicate with patients about sexuality.

References

Aggleton P. and Chalmers H. (1986). Model choice. *Senior Nurse* 5 (5/6), November/December: 18–20.

Austin R. (1977). Sex and Gender in the Future of Nursing. *Nursing Times*, Occasional Papers; (i) 73 (34): 113–16; (ii) 73(35): 117–19.

Barnett K. (1972a). A survey of the current utilisation of touch by health team personnel with hospitalised patients. *International Journal of Nursing Studies* 9:195–209.

Barnett K. (1972b). A theoretical construct of the concepts of touch as they relate to nursing. *Nursing Research* 21(2) March–April: 102–10.

Barrett M. (1980). *Women's Oppression Today*. London: New Left Books and Verso.

de Beauvoir S. (1975). *The Second Sex*. Harmondsworth: Penguin.

Beer C., Jeffery R. and Munyard T. (1983). *Gay Workers: Trade Unions and the Law*. London: NCCL.

Benn M. (1985). Isn't sexual harassment really about masculinity? *Spare Rib* 156:6–8.

Boerigger J. (1973). *What You Always Wanted to Know about Sex in Uniform But Were Afraid to Ask*. London: Capri Publishers.

Bolton G. (1980). Preparing for the next decade. *Nursing Times*, January 3: 26–28.

Brake M. (1982). Sexuality as praxis—a consideration of the contribution of sexual theory to the process of sexual being. *Human Sexual Relations: A Reader*. Harmondsworth: Penguin.

Brandes S. (1981). Like wounded stags: male sexual ideology in an Andalusian town. In *Sexual Meanings* (S. Ortner and H. Whitehead, eds). Cambridge: Cambridge University Press.

British Medical Journal (1986). Editorial: Risk of AIDS to health care workers. *British Medical Journal* 292 (6522): 711–12.

Brown E. (1966). Nursing and patient care. In *The Nursing Profession* (F. Davis ed.). Chichester: John Wiley.

Brown M. (1977). *Normal Development of Body Image*. New York: John Wiley.

Brown R., Haddox V., Posada A., Rubio A. (1972). Social and psychological adjustment following pelvic exenteration. *American Journal of Obstetrics and Gynaecology* **114**:162.

Cant B. (1985). Pain in the arse. *New Statesman* **110**(2851): 36–7.

Capra F. (1983). *The Tao of Physics: An Exploration of the Parallels between Modern Physics and Eastern Mysticism*. London: Flamingo.

Carter A. (1982). *The Sadeian Woman*. London: Virago.

Chapman C. (1978). A philosophy of nursing practice and education. *Nursing Times* **74**(8): 303–5.

Commission on Nursing Education (1985). *The Education of Nurses: A New Dispensation*. London: Royal College of Nursing.

Cooper L. (1985). *The Happy Ward*. London: Mills & Boon.

Coward R. (1984). *Female Desire: Women's Sexuality Today*. London: Paladin.

Craik J. (1979). Reflections on the Feminine. *Cambridge Anthropology* **5**(3):77–142.

Department of Health and Social Security (1986). *Guidance for Surgeons, Anaesthetists, Dentists and their Teams in Dealing with Patients Infected with HTLV III*. AIDS Booklet 3. London: DHSS.

Dewhurst J. (ed.) (1981). *Integrated Obstetrics and Gynaecology for Post-Graduates*. Oxford: Blackwell Scientific.

Dingwall R. (1979). The place of men in nursing. In *Readings in Nursing* (M. Colledge and D. Jones, eds). Edinburgh: Churchill Livingstone.

Dixon B. (1985). Unflattering reflections. *New Scientist*. October 24(1979):54.

Dolan M. (1985). An Eternal Flame. *Nursing 1985* **15**(1):20.

Eardley A. and Thornton M. (1976). Post-surgical problems. *Nursing Mirror* **142**(5):58–9.

Easlea B. (1981). *Science and Sexual Oppression: Patriarchy's Confrontation with Woman and Nature*. London: Weidenfeld & Nicolson.

Edwards G. (1984). Breaking a Tradition. *Nursing Mirror* **159**(10): 18–20.

Ehrenreich B. and English D. (1973). *Witches, Midwives and Nurses: A History of Women Healers*. London: Writers & Readers.

Eichenbaum L. and Orbach S. (1983). *What Do Women Want?* London: Michael Joseph.

Emerson J. (1971). Behaviour in private places: sustaining definitions of reality in gynaecological examinations. In *Recent Sociology* (Number 2) (H. Dreitzel ed.) New York: Collier Macmillan.

Evans T. (1983) *Griffiths: "The Right Prescription"*. London: Chartered Inst. Public Finance & Assoc. Health Service Treasurers.

Fagin C. and Diers D. (1984). Nursing as metaphor. *International Nursing Review* **31**(1): 16–17.

Farabaugh N. (1984). Do nurse educators promote burnout? *International Nursing Review* **31**(2): 47–52.

Fisher S. and Cleveland S. (1958). *Body Image and Personality*. New York: von Nostrand.

Fontaine K. (1976). Human sexuality: faculty knowledge and attitudes. *Nursing Outlook* **24**(3): 174–6.

Foucault M. (1973). *The Birth of the Clinic: An Archaelogy of Medical Perception*. London: Tavistock.

Gagnon J. and Simon W. (1973). *Sexual Conduct: The Social Sources of Human Sexuality*. Chicago: Aldine Publishing Co.

Goffman E. (1961) *Asylums Essays on the Social Situation of Mental Patients and Other Inmates*. New York: Anchor.

Glover J. (1985). *Human Sexuality in Nursing Care*. London: Croom Helm.

Goldwyn E. (1979). The Fight to be Male. *The Listener*. May 24, pp. 709–11.

Goodykoontz L. (1979). Touch: Attitudes and Practice. *Nursing Forum* **xviii**(1): 5–17.

Gordon D. (1986). Models of clinical expertise in American nursing practice. *Social Science and Medicine* **22**(9): 953–61.

Gove W. (1984). Gender differences in mental and physical illness: the effects of fixed roles and nurturant roles. *Social Science and Medicine* **19**(2): 77–91.

Gow K. (1982) *How Nurses Emotions Affect Patient Care: Self Studies by Nurses*. New York: Springer Publishing Co.

Groff B. (1984). The trouble with male nursing. *American Journal of Nursing* **84**(1): 62–3.

Groth A., Burgess A., Holstram L. (1977). Rape: Power, anger and sexuality. *American Journal of Psychiatry* **134**:1239–43.

Hadjifotiou N. (1983). *Women and Harassment at Work*. London: Pluto Press.

Hall E. (1966). *The Hidden Dimension: Man's Use of Space in Public and Private*. London: The Bodley Head.

Hamilton A. (1976). The problems of the arthritic patient. *Nursing Mirror* **142**:54–5.

Helman C. (1978). Feed a cold, starve a fever: Folk models of infection in an English suburban community and their relation to medical treatment. *Culture, Medicine and Psychiatry:* **2**:107–37.

Henderson V. (1966). *The Nature of Nursing*. New York: Macmillan.

Henley M. (1973). Status and sex: Some touching observations. *Bulletin of the Psychosomatic Society* **2**(2): 91–3.

Hesford A., Bhanji S. (1986). Sexual dysfunction in women. *Nursing Times* **82**(14): 49–51.

Hite S. (1977). *The Hite Report: A Nationwide Study on Female Sexuality*. London: Talmy Franklin Ltd.

Hite, S. (1981). *The Hite Report on Male Sexuality*. London: Macdonald.

Hoban R. (1976). *Kleinzeit*. London: Picador.

Holder S. (1973). Rediscovering the patient. *Nursing Times*, October 4: 1275–7.

Hollingworth S. (1985). *Preparation for Change: Preparing Nurse Tutors in Initial Training for a Change to Nursing Process*. London: Royal College of Nursing.

Hunt J., Marks-Maran D. (1986) (2nd ed.). *Nursing Care Plans: The Nursing Process at Work*. Chichester: John Wiley.

Jenkins R, Clare A. (1985). Women and Mental Illness. *British Medical Journal* **291** (6508): 1521–2.

Jewson N. (1976). The disappearance of the sick-man from medical cosmology, 1770–1870. *Sociology* **10**:225–44.

Jones J. (1985). Subordination out of choice? Letter to *Nursing Times* **81**(4): 14.

Jones M. (1985). Too political. Letter to *Nursing Mirror* **160**(20): 16.

Jones R. (1983). *Physics as Metaphor*. London: Abacus.

Jourard S. (1971). *The Transparent Self*. New York: van Nostrand Reinhold.

Kalisch B., Kalisch P., Scobey M. (1983). *Images of the Nurse on Television*. New York: Springer Publishing Co.

Kaplan H. (1974). *The New Sex Therapy*. London: Baillière Tindall.

Kershaw B., Salvage J. (eds) (1986). *Models for Nursing*. Chichester: John Wiley.

Kesey K. (1973). *One Flew Over the Cuckoo's Nest*. London: Picador.

Kitson A. (1985). Educating for quality. *Senior Nurse* **3** (4): 11–16.

Kneisl C., Wilson H. (1984). *Handbook of Psychosocial Nursing Care*. Menlo Park, California: Addison-Wesley Publishing.

Krajicek M. (1982). Developmental disability and human sexuality. *Nursing Clinics of North America* **17**(3): 377–85.

Kreuger C. (1978). Good Girls—Bad Girls. In *Readings in the Sociology of Nursing*. (R. Dingwall and J. McIntosh, eds) Edinburgh: Churchill Livingstone.

Krieger D. (1975). Therapeutic touch: The imprimatur of nursing. *American Journal of Nursing* **75**(5): 784–7.

Lear M. (1981). *Heartsounds*. London: Arrow Books.

Lieven E. (1981). 'If it's natural, we can't change it.' *Women in Society: Interdisciplinary Essays*. (Cambridge Women's Studies Group.) London: Virago.

Lion E. (1982). Human sexuality: a concept basic to nursing. *Human Sexuality in Nursing Process*. New York: John Wiley.

Mace, D., Bannerman R., Burton J. (eds) (1974). *The Teaching of Human Sexuality in Schools for Health Professionals*. Geneva: World Health Organization.

McAllister H. (1985). Aspects of AIDS. Letter to *Nursing Times*, **81**(21): 14.

McCarey J. (1973). *Human Sexuality*. Cincinnati: van Nostrand Reinhold.

McCurdy J. (1982). Power *is* a nursing issue. In *Socialisation, Sexism and Stereotyping: Women's Issues in Nursing* (J. Muff, ed.). St Louis: C. V. Mosby Co.

McFarlane J. (1985). Nursing—images and reality. *Nursing Mirror*, **160**(1): 16–18.

McFarlane J. (1986). The value of models for care. In *Models for Nursing* (B. Kershaw and J. Salvage, eds). Chichester: John Wiley.

Macintyre S. (1976). 'Who wants babies?'—The social construction of instincts. In *Sexual Divisions and Society: Process and Change* (D. Barker and S. Allen, eds) London: Tavistock.

McKeighen R. (1978). Drives, differences and deviations. *Human Sexuality for Health Professionals*. Philadelphia: W.B. Saunders.

Mackintosh, M. (1981). The sexual division of labour and the subordination of women. In *Of Marriage and the Market* (K. Young, C. Wolkowitz and R. McCullagh, eds) London: CSE Books.

McLaren A. (1984). *Reproductive Rituals: The Perception of Fertility from the Sixteenth to the Nineteenth Century*. London: Methuen.

MacRae D. (1975). The body and social metaphor. In *The Body as a Medium of Expression* (J. Benthall and T. Polhemus, eds). London: Allen Lane.

MacRae I., Henderson G. (1975). Sexuality and irreversible health limitations. Nursing Clinics of North America **10**(3): 587–97.

Maddock J. (1975). Sexual health and sexual health care. *Postgraduate Medicine* **58**:52–8.

Masters W., Johnson V. (1966). *Human Sexual Response*. Boston: Little, Brown & Co.

Merleau-Ponty M. (1962). *Phenomonology of Perception*. London: Routledge & Kegan Paul.

Miller H. (1965) *Sexus*. New York: Grove Press.

Miller S. (1984). Recognising the sexual health care needs of hospitalised patients. *Canadian Nurse* **80**(3): 43–6.

Millet K. (1977). *Sexual Politics*. London: Virago.

Mitchell T. (1984). 'Is nursing any business of doctors?' A simple guide to the nursing process. *British Medical Journal* **288** (6412): 216–19.

Money J., Ehrhardt A. (1972). *Man and Woman, Boy and Girl*. Baltimore: Johns Hopkins University Press.

Montagu A. (1978). (2nd ed.) *Touching: The Human Significance of the Skin*. New York: Harper & Row.

Muff J. (1982). Handmaiden, battle-ax, whore: an exploration into the fantasies, myths and stereotypes about nurses. *Socialisation, Sexism and Stereotyping: Women's Issues in Nursing*. St Louis: C. V. Mosby Co.

Newton L. (1981). In Defense of the Traditional Nurse. *Nursing Outlook* **29**(6): 348–54.

Norwell N. (1986). Bible has comfort for the cold. *General Practitioner* March 14:21.

Nursing Times (1980). A uniform fit for the 80s. *Nursing Times* **76**(21): 896–7.

Nursing Times News (1985). Nurses with children suffer in NHS career stakes. *Nursing Times* **81**(28): 8.

Nuttall P. (1983). Male takeover or female giveaway? *Nursing Times* **79**(2): 10–11.

Oakley A. (1972). *Sex, Gender and Society*. London: Temple Smith.

Oakley A. (1984). The importance of being a nurse. *Nursing Times* **80**(50): 24–7.

Olesen V., Whittaker E. (1968). *The Silent Dialogue: A Study in the Social Psychology of Professional Socialisation*. San Francisco: Jossey-Bass Inc.

Orbach S. (1982). *Fat is a Feminist Issue: A Programme to Conquer Compulsive Eating*. New York: Berkley Books.

Ortner S., Whitehead H. (1981). Introduction: Accounting for Sexual Meanings. *Sexual Meanings: The Cultural Construction of Gender and Sexuality*. Cambridge: Cambridge University Press.

Patton C. (1985). *Sex and Germs: The Politics of AIDS*. Boston: South End Press.

Pearson A. (1983). *The Clinical Nursing Unit*. London: Heinemann.

Pearson A., Vaughan B. (1986). *Nursing Models for Practice*. London: Heinemann.

Person E. (1980). Sexuality as the mainstay of identity: psychoanalytic perspectives. In *Women—Sex and Sexuality* (C. Stimpson and E. Person, eds). Chicago: University of Chicago Press.

Pfeffer N., Woollett A. (1983). *The Experience of Infertility*. London: Virago.

Playboy (1983). Women in white. *Playboy* **30**(11): 88–97, 224.

Plummer K. (1982). Symbolic Interactionism and Sexual Conduct: An Emergent Perspective. In *Human Sexual Relations: A Reader in Human Sexuality* (M. Brake, ed.). Harmondsworth: Penguin.

Pongoncheff E. (1979). The gay patient. *Registered Nurse* **42**:46–52.

Postal S. (1965). *Body image and identity: a comparison of Kwakiutl and Hopi*. *American Anthropologist* 67: 455–62.

Raphael-Leff J. (1986). Infertility: diagnosis or life sentence? *British Journal of Sexual Medicine*, January: 28–9.

Reuhl S. (1983). Sexual Theory and Practice: Another Double Standard. In *Sex and Love: New Thoughts on Old Contradictions* (S. Cartledge, J. Ryan, eds). London: Women's Press.

Rickford F. (1983). No more sleeping beauties and frozen boys. In *The Left and The Erotic* (E. Phillips, ed.). London: Lawrence & Wishart.

Riley E. (1986). Sex after a CVA *British Journal of Sexual Medicine*, January:18.

Roberts H. (1985). *The Patient Patients: Women and their Doctors*. London: Pandora Press.

Root J. (1984). *Pictures of Women: Sexuality*. London: Pandora Press.

Roper N., Logan W., Tierney A. (1985) (2nd ed.). *The Elements of Nursing*. Edinburgh: Churchill Livingstone.

Rosen J. & Jones K. (1972). The male nurse. *New Society* **68:**493–4.

RCN (1986a) *Memorandum on the Implementation of the Griffiths Report in the National Health Service*. London: RCN.

RCN (1986b). *Nursing Guidelines on the Management of Patients in Hospital and the Community Suffering from AIDS*. London: RCN.

Sacks O. (1984). *A Leg To Stand On*. London: Duckworth.

Salmon Committee (1966). *Report of the Committee on Senior Nursing Staff*. London: HMSO.

Salvage J. (1982). Angles, not Angels. *The Health Services*, September 3: 12–13.

Salvage J. (1985). *The Politics of Nursing*. London: Heinemann Nursing.

Sanderson E. (1985). Nursing Patience. *Lampada* **4:**36–7.

Savage J. (1982). No sex please Mrs Smith. *Nursing Mirror* **154**(7): 28–32.

Scully D., Bart P. (1978). A funny thing happened on the way to the orifice: women in gynaecology textbooks. In *The Cultural Crisis of Modern Medicine* (J. Ehrenreich, ed.) New York: Monthly Review Press.

Segal L. (1983). Sensual uncertainty, or why the clitoris is not enough. In *Sex and Love: New Thoughts on Old Contradictions* (S. Cartledge, J. Ryan, eds). London: Women's Press.

Shore B. (1981). Sexuality and gender in Samoa: conceptions and missed conceptions. In *Sexual Meanings*. (S. Ortner and H. Whitehead, eds) (ibid).

Singleton C. (1986). Biological and social explanations of sex-role stereotyping. In *The Psychology of Sex Roles*. (Hargreaves D., Colley A., eds). London: Harper & Row.

Stein L. (1978). The doctor–nurse game. In *Readings in the Sociology of Nursing* (R. Dingwall, J. McIntosh, eds). Edinburgh: Churchill Livingstone.

Stone L. (1977). *The Family, Sex and Marriage in England, 1500–1800*. Harmondsworth: Harper Colophon Books (Penguin).

Strathern M. (1976). An anthropological perspective. In *Exploring Sex Differences* (B. Lloyd, J. Archer, eds). London: Academic Press.

Strauss A. (1966). The structure and ideology of American nursing: an interpretation. In *The Nursing Profession: Five Sociological Essays*. (F. Davis, ed.) New York: John Wiley.

Szasz S. (1982). The tyranny of uniforms. In *Socialisation, Sexism and Stereotyping*. (J. Muff, ed.) (ibid).

Terrence Higgins Trust 1985 (2nd ed.) AIDS and HTLV III: Medical Briefing.

Thompson D., Cordle C. (1986). Sexual Counselling Following Myocardial Infarction. *British Journal of Sexual Medicine*, January: 16–17.

Tschudin V. (1985). Warding off a crisis. *Nursing Times* **81**(38): 45–6.

Tschudin V. (1985/6) A fine balance. *Lampada* **6**:20–22.

Ujhely G. (1979). Touch: reflections and perceptions. *Nursing Forum:* **xviii**(1): 18–33.

Uren R. (1980). *Nurse Foster*. London: Mills & Boon.

Versluysen M. (1980). Old wives' tales? Women healers in English history. In *Rewriting Nursing History* (C. Davies, ed.). London: Croom Helm.

Webb, C. (1985a). *Sexuality, Nursing and Health*. Chichester: John Wiley.

Webb C. (1985b). Teaching sexuality in the curriculum. *Senior Nurse* **3**(5): 10–12.

Whatley M. (1986). Integrating sexuality issues into the nursing curriculum. *Journal of Sex Education and Therapy*. **12**(2): 23–26.

Whitehead H. (1981). The bow and the burden strap: a new look at institutionalised homosexuality in native North America. In *Sexual Meanings* (Ortner and Whitehead, eds.) (ibid).

Whitley M. (1978). Seduction and the hospitalised patient. *Journal of Nursing Education* **17**(6): 34–9.

Whittaker E., Olesen V. (1978). The faces of Florence Nightingale: functions of the heroine legend in an occupational sub-culture. In *Readings in the Sociology of Nursing* (R. Dingwall, J. McIntosh, eds). Edinburgh: Churchill Livingstone.

Williams K. (1978). Ideologies of nursing: their meanings and implications. In *Readings in the Sociology of Nursing* (R. Dingwall, J. McIntosh, eds) (ibid).

Wilmer V. (1981). No sex please, you're female. *Time Out*, January 23:5.

Woods N. (1984). (3rd ed.). *Human Sexuality in Health and Illness*. St Louis: C. V. Mosby.

World Health Organization (1975). *Education and Treatment in Human Sexuality: The Training of Health Professionals*. Technical Report Series No 572. Geneva: WHO.

Wright Steve (1985). It's all right in theory ... *Nursing Times* **81**(34): 19–20.

Wright Steve (1986). Developing and using a nursing model. In *Models for Nursing* (Kershaw and Salvage, eds) (ibid).

Wright Susannah (1985) Conspiracy of silence. *Nursing Mirror* **160**(20): 47–8.

Yeaworth R., Friedman J. (1975). Sexuality in later life. *Nursing Clinics of North America* **10**(3): 565–74.

Index